Health Ministry
Advice for Everyone

Deborah Patterson

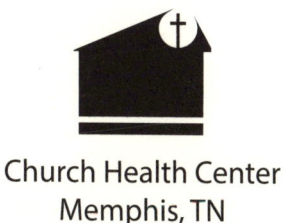

Church Health Center
Memphis, TN

About the Church Health Center

The Church Health Center seeks to reclaim the church's biblical commitment to care for our bodies and our spirits. Long recognized as a national model for serving the uninsured, the Center has spent years connecting people of faith and their congregations with quality health resources and educational experiences. To learn more about the Center, visit ChurchHealthCenter.org. To learn more about our magazine on health ministry, *Church Health Reader*, visit CHreader.org.

Health Ministry Advice for Everyone
© 2014 Deborah Patterson

The Scripture quotations contained herein are from the New Revised Standard Version Bible, copyright 1989, Division of Christian Education of the National Council of the Churches of Christ in the United States of America, and are used by permission. All rights reserved.

ISBN: 978-1-62144-042-0

Printed in the United States of America.

The Church Health Center is proud to publish this resource using recycled materials.

Cover Design: Rachel Davis

Layout and Design: Rachel Davis and Lizy Heard

Please feel free to copy and distribute this resource to your congregation or community.

*To faith community nurses and health
ministers all around the world,
and to my beloved family.*

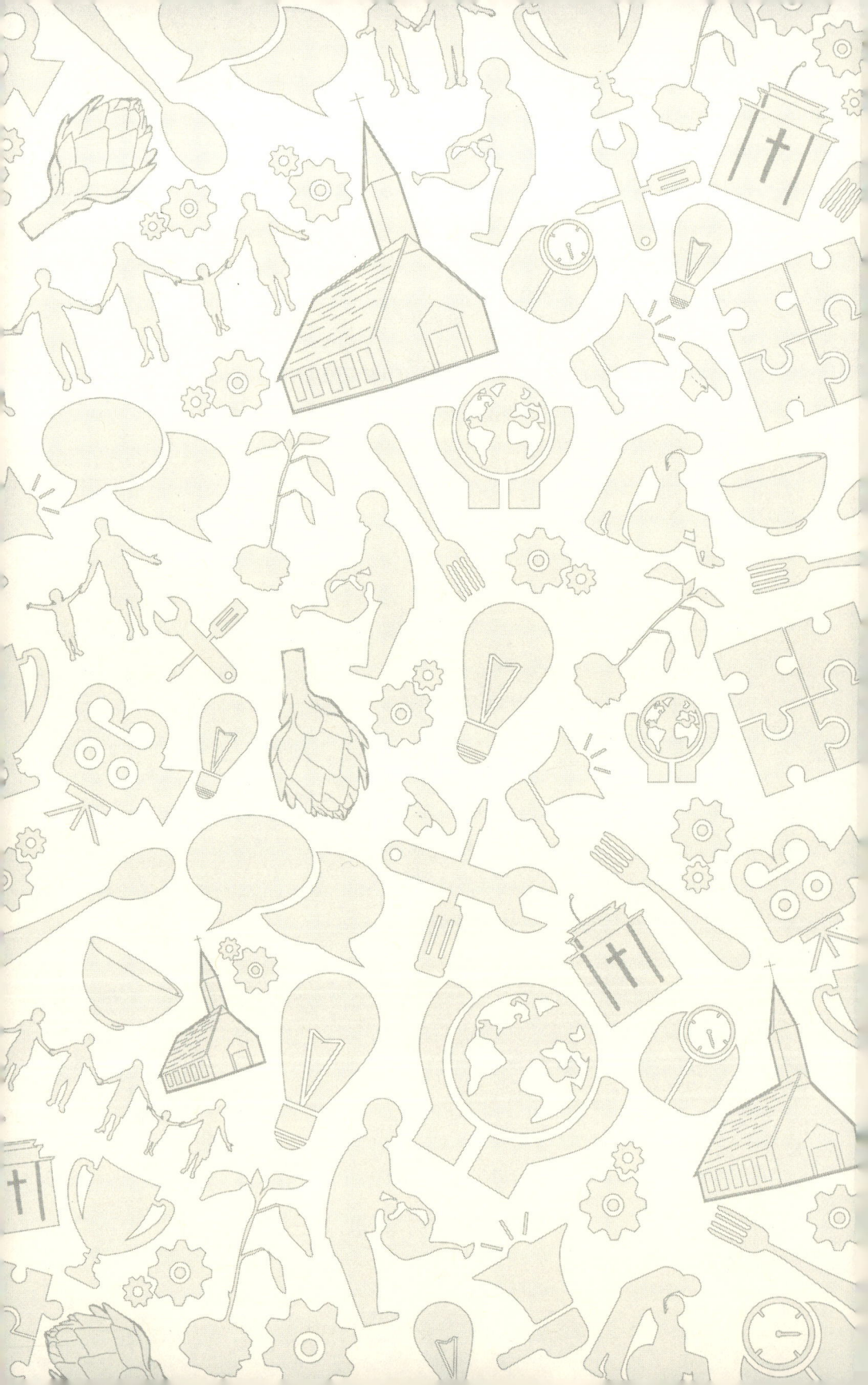

Table of Contents

Introduction	9
Chapter 1 : The Basics	13
Starting a Health Ministry	14
Small Congregations	16
Getting Started as a Health Minister	18
Top 10 Ideas for Congregations	20
Book Recommendations	22
Chapter 2: Tools for Ministry	25
Health Ministry Sunday	26
Newsletter Features	28
Communicating with Your Congregation	30
Going Deeper in Health Ministry	32
Ministry beyond the Church Walls	34
National Health Observances	36
Accessibility	38
Facing Pushback	40
Health Posters	42
Health Concerns in Worship	44
Health Ministry Sunday	46
Finding an FCN	48
Health Committee	50
Chapter 3: Promote Wellness	53
Exercise Program	54
Walking Program	56
Clergy Health	58
Healthy Meetings	60
Church Gardens	62
Healthier Coffee Hour	64
$15 Coffee Hour	66
Snack Ideas	68
Healthy Holidays	70
Spiritual Health	72

Chapter 4: Children, Youth, and Families — 75
- Children's Health — 76
- Childhood Obesity — 78
- Teen Obesity — 80
- Intergenerational Ministry — 82
- Online Safety for Teens — 84
- Advocating Public Policy — 86
- Domestic Violence — 88
- Just-in-Case Bags — 90
- Miscarriage — 92
- Adoption — 94
- Pregnancy — 96
- Eating Disorders — 98

Chapter 5: Medical Issues, Education and Prevention — 101
- Prayers for Medical Procedures — 102
- Surgery Support — 104
- Fall Prevention — 106
- Sleep Education — 108
- Funding an AED — 110
- Using an AED — 112
- Blood Pressure — 114
- Heart Disease — 116
- Foot Care Clinic — 118
- Cancer Programs — 120
- Stress Education — 122
- Mental Health — 124
- Advance Directives — 126

Chapter 6: Community Engagement — 129
- Health Disparities — 130
- Health Care Missions — 132
- Starting a Dental Clinic — 134
- Blood Drives — 136
- Cooling Center — 138
- Veteran Support — 140
- Housing — 142
- Senior Housing — 144
- Healthy Food Pantry — 146

Chapter 7: Church Life and Activities — 149
   Movie Nights — 150
   Fundraisers — 152
   Quilting — 154
   Presenting Prayer Shawls — 156
   Choir — 158
   Labyrinths — 160
   Chronic Illness Support Groups — 162
   Healing and Hymns — 164

Chapter 8: Congregational Care — 167
   Dementia — 168
   Hoarding — 170
   Loneliness — 172
   Memory Loss Support — 174
   Elder Abuse — 176
   Breast Cancer — 178
   Grieving Congregations — 180
   After-Death Paperwork — 182
   Caregiver Support — 184

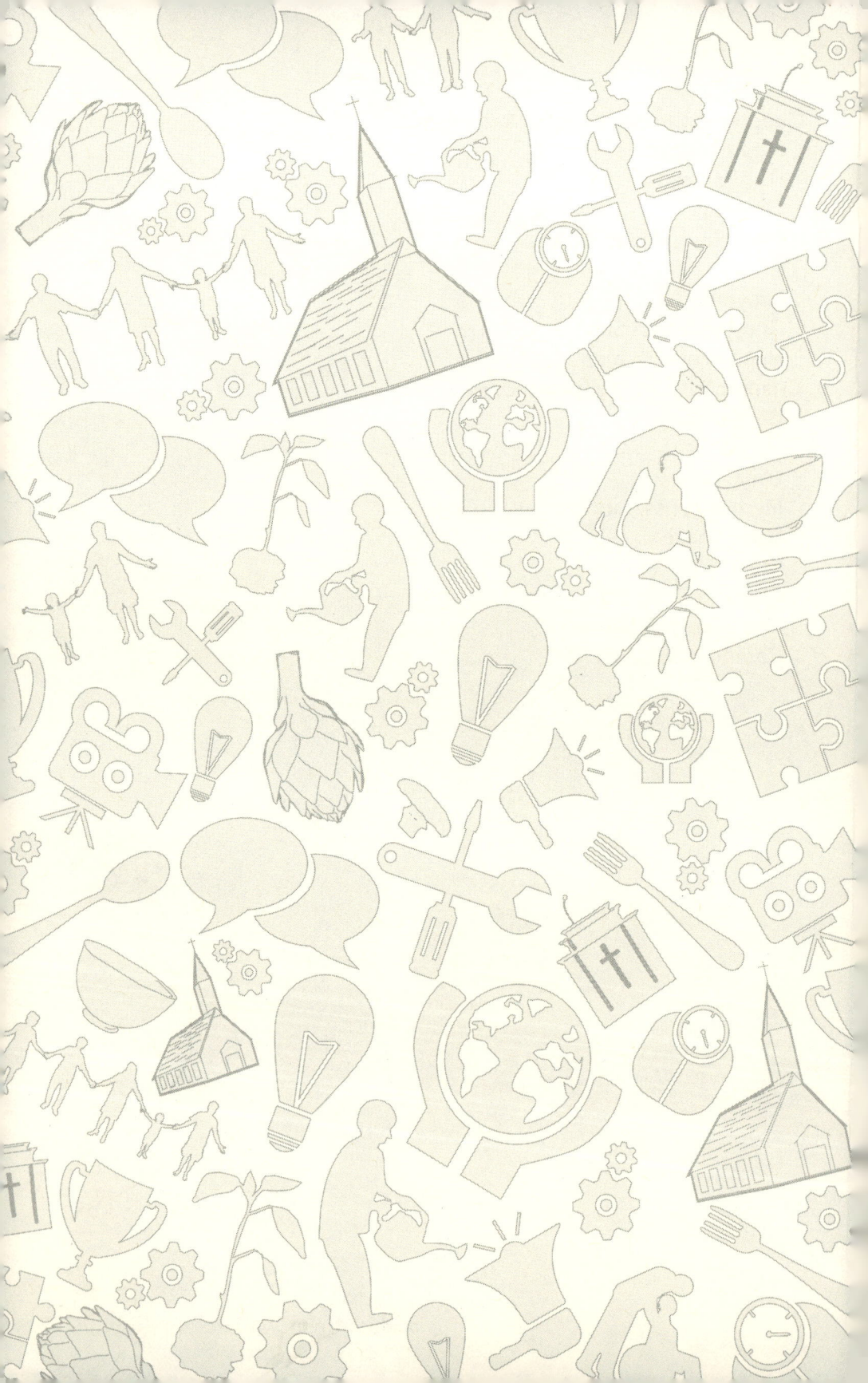

Introduction

A few years back, the Church Health Center kindly asked if I would consider writing a monthly advice column on questions about health ministry. I had served for a number of years as the executive director of the International Parish Nurse Resource Center, whose programs became part of the Church Health Center in 2011. When the column began, I was serving as the executive director of Northwest Parish Nurse Resource Center.

Not being a health professional, but rather a clergyperson, I relied heavily on the expertise of the parish nurses and other health care providers. They helped me learn about the wide variety of innovative ways to multiply the limited resources of a faith community to serve the wider community in all things health-related. Health education, health counseling, resource referral, health care advocacy, health literacy, developing support groups, and serving various age groups and health conditions were just some of the issues that came up over the years.

This work is not limited to health care professionals. Rev. Dr. Granger Westberg, the founder of faith community nursing and leader in health ministry, knew that the call to "preach, teach, and heal" is extended to all in the church. Lay people play a significant role in the delivery of health-related services in a congregation, from helping with program logistics, to visiting the sick, to helping make a home more safe, to cooking healthy food—the list of ways to participate in health ministry is endless! In fact, there were so many questions that the monthly column soon turned into a weekly column. What you hold in your hands is a compilation of many of those pieces.

So, with thanks to the Church Health Center, to the health care professionals who generously shared their best practices and hard-earned knowledge about health ministry, particularly the Deaconess Parish Nurses in the St. Louis area, the parish nurses affiliated with Northwest Parish Nurse Ministries, and the many networks of parish nurses around the world now affiliated with the Church Health Center, I offer my thanks as we seek together to serve God through this unfolding form of ministry.

I hope that this book provides not only some useful advice, culled from these many voices, but also inspiration for health and wellness initiatives in your congregation and community. I wish you the best in your endeavors in healing ministry.

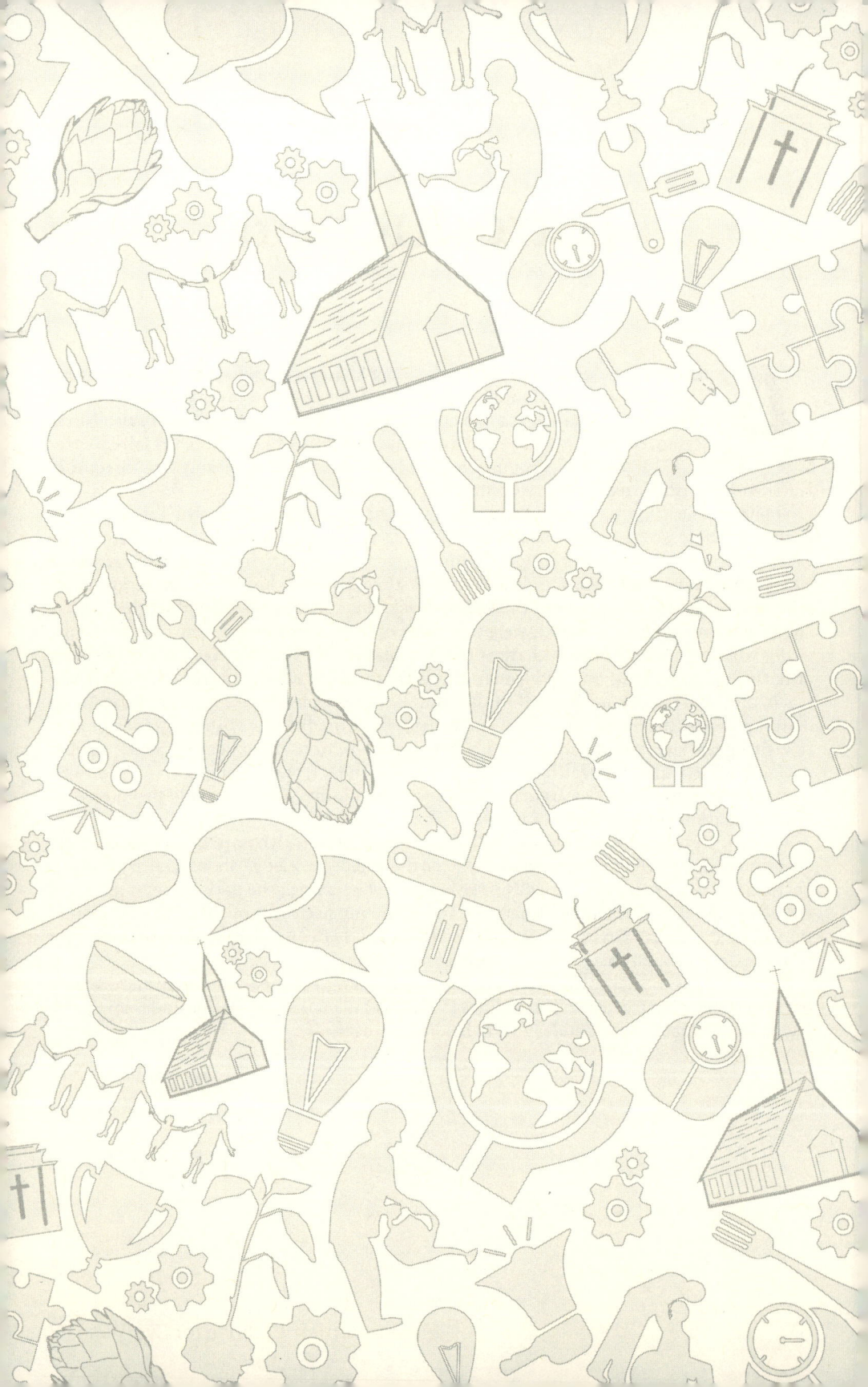

Acknowledgements

Without John Shorb's willingness to try new things, this book or the columns that preceded it would not exist. To John, my heartfelt thanks for your encouragement and for your modeling of a life balancing ministry and art.
The Church Health Center is filled with many people who make an incredible difference each day, and they are all an inspiration: Rev. Scott Morris, MD, Rev. Stacy Smith, Sarah Ranson, Katora Campbell and, of course, Maureen Daniels, with whom I worked closely in St. Louis for many years. As my kids would say, y'all rock!

Thanks to Sandy Madsen, Karen Wright, Jeanne Brotherton, Dotty Marston, Debbi Saint, and other coordinators at NPNM for letting me learn so much from you. And thanks to the Deaconess Parish Nurses—you know who you are—who continue to be an inspiration, under the able leadership of Rev. Donna Pupillo, RN. Alvyne Rethemeyer, who started in this field one week before I did at Deaconess Health System, you are a blessing. And to the family of Rev. Dr. Granger Westberg, and to Ann Solari-Twadell, PhD, thanks beyond measure for your wisdom and grace.

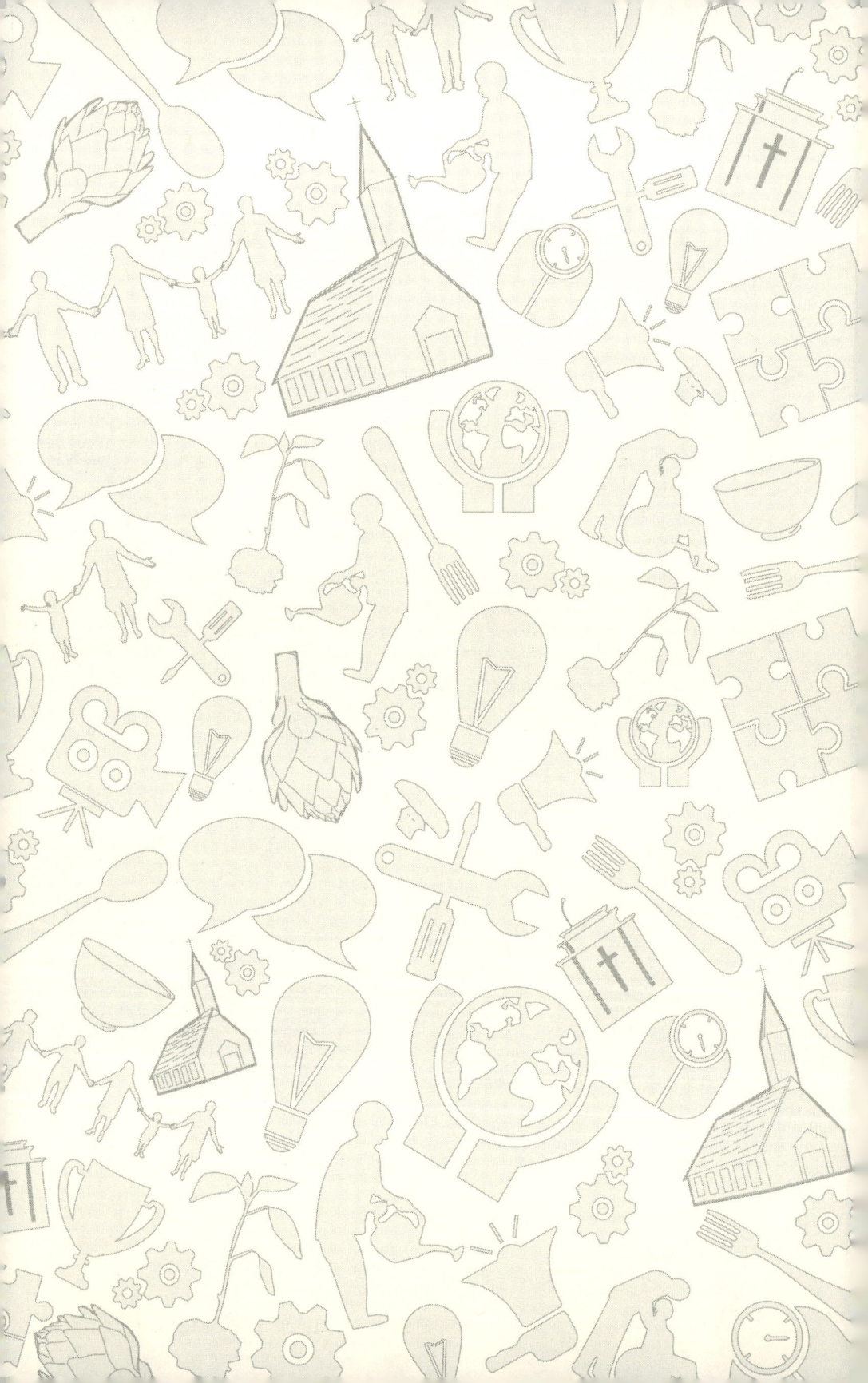

CHAPTER 1

The Basics

Starting a Health Ministry

QUESTION
How should a church start a health ministry?

If your congregation is starting a health ministry, you are in good company! Growing numbers of churches are reclaiming the call they have not only to preach and to teach, but also to heal.

Faith communities started most of the hospitals, nursing schools, and medical schools around the world. The church, however, has been modest as it redefined its role in health care, overshadowed by the explosion of knowledge and technology in health care since the founding of those institutions.

For the last few decades, the healing ministry of congregations has often been limited to praying for and visiting the sick. There is nothing wrong with those activities, but a church can do much more! And health ministry can be life-transforming for those who participate when the load is shared. An active health ministry is a call to the body of Christ.

A good way to begin is to ask some questions about health ministry, such as the following:

- How has the congregation historically participated in healing ministries?
- What does Scripture say about health and healing? Was this just something for Jesus, or do we have a role?
- What are the pressing health needs in the church? In the wider community?
- What are the assets of the church? Are there health professionals, teachers, and other supporters available?
- What kinds of health ministry would the church like to see? Programs for new parents, for individuals without access to health care, exercise programs, visitation programs?

Then, get started! Here are three ways to start:

1. Launch a user-friendly, easy to implement exercise or wellness program. There are many faith-based models, including *Walk and Talk*, *Walk to Jerusalem*, *Get My People Going!*, among others.

2. Put a health tip in each bulletin or newsletter, or on a bulletin board at church, or on a bathroom wall. Most hospitals will provide blurbs, posters, or articles on many topics of interest. There are a host of national health organizations that will give you material (much is web-based). Some organizations have material specifically for faith-based organizations, such as the International Parish Nurse Resource Center at the Church Health Center.

3. Call upon the experts in your congregation and community. Most hospitals and other health organizations have speakers' bureaus and can send someone to speak with your church groups for a modest fee (or free). If you have a registered nurse who is willing to serve as a faith community nurse (either in a paid or unpaid position), encourage her or him to go take a *Foundations in Faith Community Nursing* course. This course presents the theory and practice of this nursing specialty. Part of the course includes information on getting started.

Don't delay! The fields are white unto harvest, and God is calling *you*!

Small Congregations

QUESTION
We don't have any health professionals in our small congregation of 150 people. Is there anything we can do to start a health ministry?

Of course there is! First of all, pull together a small health committee. Two heads are better than one, and five heads are better than two. Even a small church can have a health committee. And this health committee wouldn't need to do everything related to promoting health in a congregation. It would simply focus on asking the question, "What in health is going on?" In other words, how is holistic health reflected in the activities of the church—preaching, announcements, Sunday school classes, church council meetings, Vacation Bible School, coffee hour, prayer time, and pastoral visitation? Make health a regular part of conversations.

Practically speaking, what else could be done within a small church?

- Someone in the church might provide fruit and veggie snacks for a coffee hour or two and work with a committee to provide healthier offerings on an ongoing basis.

- Work with those who are leading Vacation Bible School to add physical activities and healthy snacks to the program (with no sugary drinks).

- Invite a local nutritionist to teach a healthy cooking class at the church for a fun activity on a cold winter's evening.

- Arrange for representatives from your local Area Agency on Aging to come and talk with folks in your congregation about services and resources available in the community.

- Arrange for a physician from your local hospital to come and talk about a specific heath topic. You could arrange for a whole series based on the national health observances, which you can find online.

- Invite a chaplain from a local hospice care center to come and talk about advance directives and the difference between palliative care and hospice care.

- Work with volunteers in your congregation to do safety checks in the homes of those who are elderly to help identify needs, such as for railings and grab bars. Make sure you are ready with a plan to meet the needs you identify, such as lining up a carpenter in your church who could install them.

- Get everyone involved in a walking program.

There are many more ideas throughout this book. Be creative to make ideas work for a congregation of your size. Experts in many communities will be glad to help when called upon. Everyone needs to play a role in health ministries.

Getting Started as a Health Minister

QUESTION
I've just begun my new role as a health minister. How do I get started?

Congratulations for your willingness to answer the call to care! I assume, since you have been called as a health minister, that you have the support of the clergy. I recommend you move quickly, if you haven't done so already, to set up a health committee with whom you can work on health ministries in your congregation. Here are some important things to remember when starting your health ministry:

- Be sure to take time to talk about the theological underpinnings for what you are doing with the clergy and your health committee. *Dust and Breath: Faith, Health, and Why the Church Should Care about Both* is a great resource for learning more.

- Expand this conversation to the entire congregation through formats such as special luncheons, adult education classes, small groups, and ministry teams. A brief presentation will get the conversation going and demonstrate that health ministry is for everyone, not just a committee.

- Keep the health ministry visible through a bulletin board you update regularly. There are lots of good, free materials available from the CDC, NIH and other governmental agencies.

- Another way to have great visibility for your ministry is to put a health tip in your church bulletin. You can find great congregational health information in a variety of places, including *Church Health Reader* (a quarterly publication also available online), your denominational health ministry programs, or through a faith community nurse.

- Don't forget your church newsletter! You can also find newsletter articles that can be reprinted from sources such as the National Women's Health Resource Center, if you credit the source.

- Partner with local health care professionals to provide services to your congregation. For example, many hospitals and other health organizations have speaker services and will be glad to provide speakers on a wide range of topics.

- Advertise your programs to the community. Your local newspaper may offer free calendar listings.

- Partner with health ministers in other congregations. See if there is a parish nurse network or other organization working with health ministry with which you can get involved.

- Consider a "ready-to-use" program you can offer through your congregation, such as *Get My People Going!* or *Faith and Health in the Bible*, both published by the Church Health Center. These two are specifically designed for use in faith communities. Other programs, such as the Chronic Disease Self-Management Program offered through Stanford University, can be implemented by health ministers who have been trained to offer the program. One good way to find these programs is by checking with your local health departments and other organizations such as the Alzheimer's Association and Arthritis Foundation.

Finally, stay in regular communication with your health committee and the clergy of your congregation by documenting what you are doing so that you can report your activity on a regular basis.

Top 10 Ideas for Congregations

QUESTION
What are your top ten ways that a congregation can improve the health of its members and community?

1. Encourage folks to spend time with each other and make sure that no one in the congregation or community suffers from what the World Health Organization says causes the highest risk for illness: loneliness.

2. Urge everyone to eat 9–13 servings of fruits and vegetables each day, and be sure to incorporate multiple fruit and vegetable options into church meals. According to the Harvard School of Public Health, "The latest dietary guidelines call for five to thirteen servings of fruits and vegetables a day…, depending on one's caloric intake. For a person who needs 2,000 calories a day to maintain weight and health, this translates into nine servings, or 4½ cups per day." Further, "compared with those in the lowest category of fruit and vegetable intake (less than 1.5 servings a day), those who averaged 8 or more servings a day were 30 percent less likely to have had a heart attack or stroke."

3. Encourage everyone to exercise 30 minutes a day. For those who are ready for a more ambitious challenge, aim for ten thousand steps a day. (Just Google *10,000 Steps* and see what you find. Amazing!)

4. Ask the congregation to stop serving foods with sugar, and encourage people to cut back on sugar-sweetened drinks and foods. Help them understand that too much sugar contributes to long-term health issues such as childhood and adult obesity, diabetes or dental health.

5. Educate everyone on the risk factors for, and warning signs of, heart attacks and strokes. Educating people about these things can save lives, since so few people really know.

6. Invite folks to support each other as they seek to change health practices, such as forming a walking group. Group support certainly has helped people deal with other challenging health issues, such as drug and alcohol abuse.

7. Support individuals and families living with mental illness by accepting them, providing education about mental illness to the congregation and community, and helping to provide access to quality mental health services. Working with the National Alliance for the Mentally Ill or Pathways to Promise are good ways to start.

8. Facilitate access to affordable housing for seniors, people with disabilities, and low-income families.

9. Find ways to protect the health of the environment by planting trees and plants, driving cars that don't use gas, supporting public transportation, and biking or walking.

10. Buy an Automated External Defibrillator (AED) and make sure folks learn how to use it. The data shows that using an AED when needed can help save lives. The American Heart Association has a course locater that uses your zip code to help you find courses in your area. These are offered through a wide variety of organizations, including hospitals, community colleges, and fire/rescue training organizations. Go online and search for "Heartsaver AED classes."

Health Ministry Advice for Everyone

Book Recommendations

QUESTION

Our congregational care team wants to learn more. What 10 books would you recommend on health ministry and faith community nursing?

If you are putting together a good library on these topics, I would pick these 10 books. They will help you gain a theological foundation for health ministry as well as give you practical perspectives that you can apply to your setting.

- *Dust and Breath: Faith, Health, and Why the Church Should Care about Both* by Kendra Hotz and Matt Matthews (2012)
- *The Parish Nurse: Providing a Minister of Health for Your Congregation* by Granger E. Westberg and Jill Westberg McNamara (1990).
- *Granger Westberg Verbatim: A Vision for Faith and Health*, edited by William Peterson (1982).
- *Health and Wellness: What Your Faith Community Can Do* by Jill Westberg McNamara (2006).
- *Deeply Woven Roots: Improving the Quality of Life in Your Community* by Gary Gunderson (1997).
- *Health, Healing and Wholeness: Engaging Congregations in Ministries of Health* by Mary Chase-Ziolek (2005).
- *God, Health and Happiness* by G. Scott Morris (2011).
- *The Leading Causes of Life* by Gary Gunderson with Larry Pray (2007).
- *The Right Road: Life Choices for Clergy* by Gwen Haalas (2004).
- *I Am The Lord Who Heals You: Reflections on Healing, Wholeness and Restoration* by G. Scott Morris (2004).

These books have encouraged me in my work in faith and health. I have also written about specific health ministry topics you may be interested in.

- *The Essential Parish Nurse: ABCs for Congregational Health Ministry* by Deborah L. Patterson (2003).
- *Health Ministries: A Primer for Clergy and Congregations* by Deborah L. Patterson (2008).
- *The Healing Word: Preaching and Teaching Health Ministry* by Deborah L. Patterson (2009).

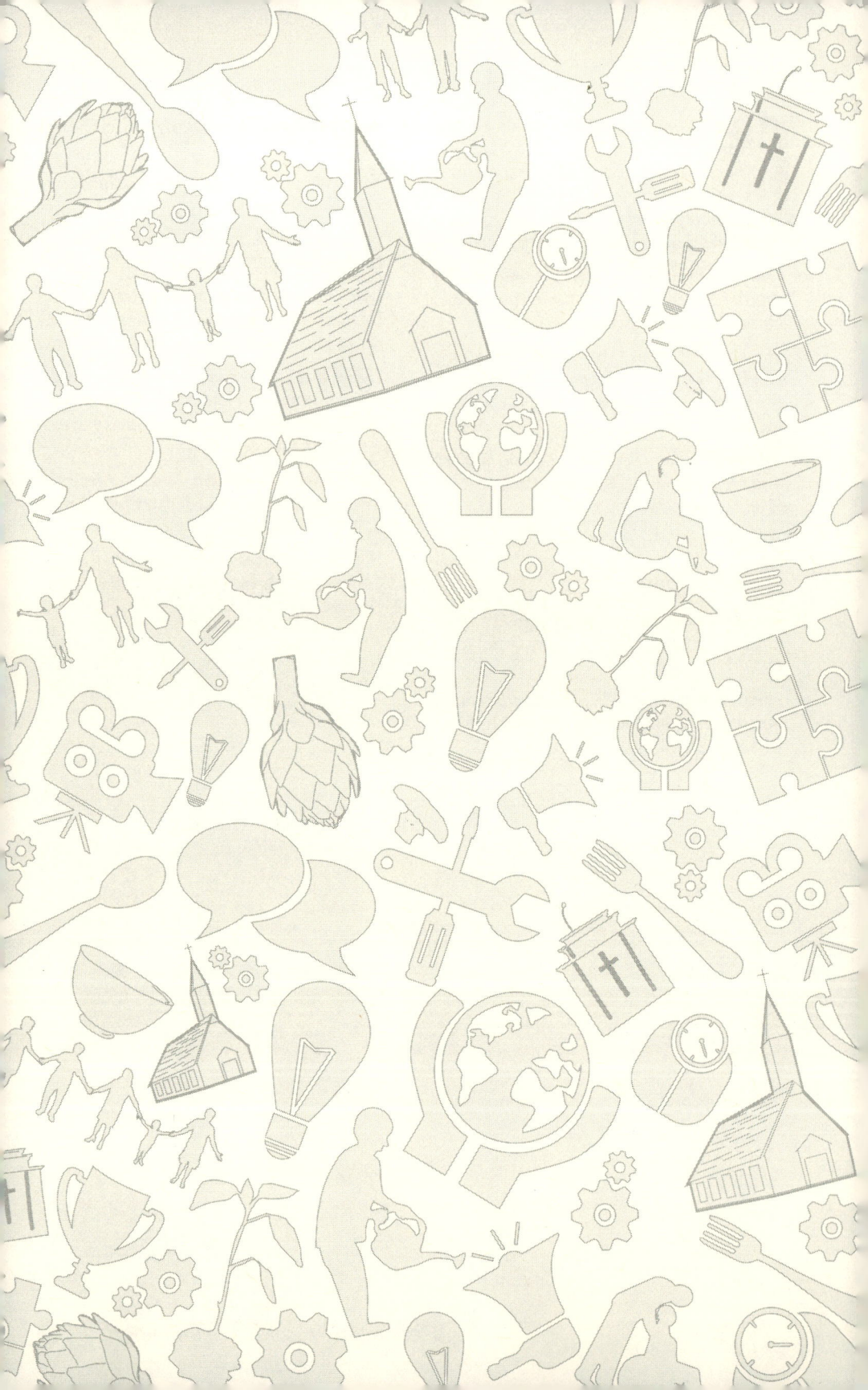

CHAPTER 2

Tools for Ministry

Health Ministry Sunday

QUESTION

My pastor has asked if our health committee could put together a Health Ministry Sunday. How should we get started on this, and when it should be held?

A health ministry Sunday is a great way to raise the visibility for the work of the health ministry committee and any faith community or parish nurse who may be a part of the ministry team.

There isn't a "Health Ministry Sunday" date designated across denominations. However, various denominations have in past years designated specific Sundays for highlighting health ministry. For example, the Presbyterian Church (USA) designated February 19, 2012 as "Health Awareness and Day of Prayer for Healing and Wholeness." The North American Division of the Seventh-day Adventist Church designated September 23, 2012 as "Let's Move Sunday." This approach to a health ministry Sunday connects with the national initiative of the same name. Check with your denomination to see if they have a health ministry Sunday and materials, or borrow from another denomination's materials.

Here are some of the elements you may want to include in a health ministry Sunday.

- Recognition of the members of the health ministry team as part of the worship service. This may also be a good time to install members of the health committee.
- Thanks for the support of the clergy for the health ministry of the congregation.
- Recognition that all members of the congregation are involved in some aspect of health ministry, from bringing healthy food for potlucks to modeling the healthy practice of singing in the choir or teaching healthy lifestyles to kids through the Christian education program.
- Hymns that lift up healing and wholeness. Ask your choir director or music leader for help.
- Plenty of time for prayer, both spoken and unspoken. You could have people write prayer requests in a special book or you may ask people to write down prayer requests to put into the offering plate. Use your imagination, but be sure to protect people's privacy.
- Some sort of ritual that denotes healing, such as lighting candles, anointing with oil, hand washing with a basin and towel, blessing of the hands, sprinkling with holy water from a branch, or foot washing. Talk with your pastor to see what might be right within your faith community's tradition. You want people to feel blessed, not uncomfortable.
- Healing music by the church musicians for the prelude, postlude, anthems and during the healing ritual, if you use one.
- Facial tissue available in the pews; sometimes this sort of service elicits the healing work of grief.
- An offering to support the health ministry of the congregation.
- A sermon on health ministry. If the pastor preaches about it, people are more likely to take it seriously.
- Healthy foods for your coffee hour, or healthy foods at a potluck following the service.

The key to success with a health ministry Sunday is to thank and recognize all who are involved, as well as to provide time and space for reflection on healing and wholeness by all. If you can get folks to see that they are all involved at some level, you will have succeeded in helping to bring the healing ministry of the church back into the core. After all, we are all together called to be the church and preach, teach, and heal.

Health Ministry Advice for Everyone

Newsletter Features

QUESTION

We would like to have a regular feature in our newsletter related to health ministry. Do you have any ideas how to start?

There is probably no better value for your investment of time in health ministry than in writing good health education articles for your congregation's newsletter. While the task might seem overwhelming, actually it is a fairly easy process that gets easier as you move forward. Here are a few tips to help you get started.

- Plan a year's worth of topics to keep you from getting stuck along the way. One good place to start might be the listing of National Health Observances at the website of the National Health Information Center to give you ideas of topics you might want to cover in a particular month.

- The Church Health Center in Memphis, Tennessee, has a digital resource called *Healthful Hints*, which has short articles and bulletin blurbs on a wide variety of topics, including National Health Observances, disease-specific topics, and specific topics for targeted group (children, seniors, women).

- Consider subscribing to a health newsletter from a medical school or school of public health as a source of up-to-date ideas and information. Harvard Medical School, Johns Hopkins, Tufts, and the University of California, Berkeley are some of the more well-known schools with health newsletters available for a modest fee. Several hospitals, such as Mt. Sinai Medical Center and Massachusetts General Hospital, have similar publications. The Center for Science in the Public Interest publishes the well-known *Nutrition Action Health Letter*, and there are scores of others.

- Many health systems have high quality health information available online without charge. For example, the Mayo Clinic website offers outstanding health information. The Nemours Children's Health System has a wealth of health information about children's health issues, including sections for kids and for teens, available through their KidsHealth.org website.

- Helpful health information is also available through national health and advocacy organizations such as the American Heart Association, the National Women's Health Center, and the Alzheimer's Association. Many of these organizations have newsletter articles you may reprint without charge as long as you credit the source. Some request that you inform them when you use their articles.

- Check out the health sections of your local newspaper and of a national newspaper as well, such as *The New York Times*. The *Times* also has several good health-related blogs with well-researched information.

- Your local library can be a great source of information. Make friends with the reference librarians and ask them to help you keep track of new health materials.

- Many local hospitals will allow residents of the area to use their libraries and sometimes will permit books and other materials to be checked out.

- Don't forget the many resources available through the National Libraries of Medicine. If you are working on a project and get stuck, give them a call. I know from experience that they are more than happy to help faith community nurses and other health ministers.

- The National Institutes of Health have more information than you could write about in a hundred lifetimes, and it is constantly being updated. They have many resources from the various institutes that you can copy for use in your congregation at no charge, including posters and articles, and both quick facts and in-depth materials for use in writing your own articles.

Make sure you include information in your church newsletter about the source of your information, how readers can learn more about a topic, and how they can reach you.

Communicating with Your Congregation

QUESTION
What are the best ways to let the congregation know what you are doing?

First of all, we know that as you tell folks about what you are doing in the congregation, you won't share any private health information about individuals; that goes without saying. But you can share the type of activities you are doing, the programs you are offering, and the numbers of people served. In addition, with the permission of the person you are helping, you can share general health concerns or prayer concerns with appropriate individuals or groups, such as the clergy, prayer circles, health team, or the congregation. If in doubt, ask for permission about what you can share, and err on the side of personal privacy.

Related to telling people about what you do, of course you are going to use the obvious ways of sharing the good news about what you are doing as a health ministry team, including:

- Sharing updates with the clergy.
- Sharing information about what the health committee is doing.
- Submitting weekly bulletin blurbs to the church secretary for inclusion in the bulletin.
- Writing a monthly newsletter article on a health issue and how people can help address the issue, either for themselves or others.
- Creating a health ministry bulletin board and keeping it updated.
- Sharing a "health minute" during announcements at church.
- Designating a "Health Ministry Sunday" at church once a year, when you recognize your many volunteers and members of your health committee.
- Submitting an annual report to your congregation about this ministry.
- Putting together small health blurbs for church e-mails.
- Collecting stories (without identifying attributes) that you can share with others. Perhaps you can use testimonials in a brochure to promote your program.

I would also, however, suggest that you are called to help spread the word to others about this ministry. Talking about what kinds of things you do will help to spread the word and make it easier for other congregations to consider this ministry. Here are some suggestions about how you can do this:

- If you work with a parish nurse coordinator at a hospital, volunteer to share some of your stories in meetings where he or she is introducing this specialty practice. Telling your stories will make his or her work so much easier! (Consider giving permission to use part of one of your stories or testimonials in a brochure about the hospital's program that they can make available in print or electronically to others.)
- Tell your pastor that you would be willing to talk about faith community nursing or health ministry at a clergy gathering if he or she would be willing to do this with you.
- Write down your stories for inclusion in a newsletter sponsored by a health ministry network with which you are affiliated. Numbers are critical, but so are stories.
- Volunteer to speak to local service groups about the work you do. Perhaps there will be some ways you identify where you can work together. Leave a one-page handout for them to share with others.
- Be sure to connect with the chaplains in the hospital where you visit patients and let them know which congregation you are affiliated with. Leave your card so that they can connect back with you.

There is great need in many places for the type of work that health ministers and faith community nurses do. Please toot your own horn and help prepare the groundwork for others to plant seeds for health ministries in their congregations.

Thanks to Karen Wright (Newport, OR), Rev. Dr. Richard Cathell (Bellingham, WA), Reen Markland (Winchester, VA), Candace Huber (Gainesville, FL), Sharon Hinton (Floydada, TX), Lee Clay (Fort Atkinson, WI), Mary McGrattan (New London, CT), Kathy Medovich (Vestal, NY) for sharing their ideas on this topic.

Going Deeper in Health Ministry

QUESTION
I want to move my congregation beyond taking blood pressure once a month. What are some good ways to go a little deeper into health ministry?

Well, first of all, good for you for taking blood pressures! According to the National Institutes of Health, about 32 percent of US adults over age 20 have hypertension (that's close to 100 million people) and many don't know it. The American Society of Hypertension has a free patient education booklet on the topic that you can download online. Another wonderful resource, *My Life Check*, is available free online through the American Heart Association.

Also, taking blood pressure is a great way to have visibility around health ministry in a congregation, particularly when it is a regular event. People know that they can go on that day to that place and find someone who will check their blood pressure, and who will listen to them. Being listened to is as important as any other part of this intervention.

Having said that, why not expand your congregation's health ministry from there? One way would be to plan a "Healthy Tasting" with small samples of healthy foods that a health committee could make and set out in little cups. Include a handout about the foods, and share the recipes and some of the information in the church bulletin, newsletter or e-mail updates.

Another idea would be to have a pharmacist come over for a "brown bag lunch." Folks bring along the medications they are on in a lunch bag, and the pharmacist privately reviews them and answers questions. While this happens, serve a healthy lunch that the youth group could sponsor to raise money for a mission trip.

Do a survey of the congregation and find out what is on their minds. Would they like a walking program, a weight-loss class, a caregiver support group? Then do a little research into these areas. There are faith-based programs and community programs to support any of these initiatives and many of them are available through denominational offices and national health organizations.

And make your health ministry programming fun! See if local businesses would be willing to give you small giveaways as incentives and participation prizes. This ministry shouldn't raise *your* blood pressure!

Ministry beyond the Church Walls

QUESTION

What is the best way to approach and organize a ministry outside the church walls?

The best way to organize a ministry outside the church walls is to first find out what is needed. Ask the members in the church what they think is needed and if possible, ask the people you hope to reach.

You already know how to find the folks in the church, so ask them what they would like to see happen. Make up a brief survey to use online through a tool like Survey Monkey, or print out copies to use on a Sunday morning. People are more likely to answer if you give them a few minutes during the announcements or ask them to stay in the pew during the postlude to do this.

One good way to reach out into the community—although it is a lot of work—is to sponsor a health fair. You can survey people who attend to find out what kind of programs they might like to see in the community.

Elizabeth Durban, who served as a parish nurse at St. Gabriel the Archangel church in St. Louis for a number of years, wrote about the health fair in *The Essential Parish Nurse*. She writes, "Health fairs are excellent projects to promote health awareness and they provide a wonderful opportunity for the parish nurse [and congregation] to reach out to the whole community." (p. 103). I recommend her excellent chapter.

Durban has had fabulous success over the years with community health fairs because she started six to nine months out and had a theme, such as "Fall into Fitness." She always included many people in the process, from public relations types to those who would be willing to solicit prizes and giveaways. They developed goals and objectives for the fair. For instance, a goal would be to provide a variety of health screenings, educational materials, and referrals to community resources. The objective would be to have three components within each booth at the fair—education, experience, and excitement. The booths were divided into three categories: awareness, screenings, and demonstrations. The floor plan was carefully planned. The committee spent a lot of effort in promoting the health fair, and often had draws such as free book bags, free haircuts, or displays from an emergency helicopter EMT team. Others who have planned carefully have had similar results.

What might come from your efforts? You might decide to fund a bus to drive folks to a free dental clinic. You might partner with a mental health provider to offer counseling on a sliding scale in your facilities. You might start an after school program to offer middle school kids (who are too old for many after school programs) the chance for physical activity and a supervised place to do their homework. Churches have done this, and you can, too!

National Health Observances

QUESTION

We would like to use the National Health Observances in planning for health education programming and activities in our congregation, but there are so many choices! Which ones should we focus on?

Looks like you found the listing of National Health Observances at the US Department of Health and Human Services's website!

Some months, like March, May, September and October, are packed with a variety of health observances, while the midwinter and summer are pretty slow indeed (even though it is important to be aware of the importance of folic acid, the only national health awareness week listed on the calendar for the entire month of January in 2012). Other big issues, such as diabetes, have to vie for attention with issues like patient safety and getting enough sleep, along with the importance of school breakfasts and poison prevention—all during the busy month of March, which is generally eclipsed by spring break anyway. What to do?

You probably already have the answer right within your congregation. Take their pulse (and their blood pressure). What issues are folks facing? If it's hypertension—and it is in most congregations as one in three adults has some level of hypertension according to the CDC—then during May, observe National High Blood Pressure education month.

If a number of folks have been diagnosed with diabetes, and you suspect that hereditary or lifestyle issues for other folks may be putting them at risk, you would probably want to observe the American Diabetes Month in November, for which the Office of Disease Prevention and Health Promotion has put together a comprehensive toolkit you can download online. In the US, more than 25 million people have diabetes, with 79 million more at risk of developing Type 2 diabetes. If not controlled, diabetes can cause serious health problems like heart disease, stroke, and blindness. People can reduce their risk by eating healthy foods, getting more exercise, and keeping their weight down, and churches are great places to socialize over healthy food and to pull together walking groups and exercise classes.

There are also National Health Observances for which many community organizations have additional resources available to support your health outreach and educational activities beyond those available on the National Health Observances website. For example, Worship in Pink is an initiative of the Susan G. Komen for the Cure, which provides resources to faith communities in Oregon and Southwest Washington to raise awareness about breast cancer.

Another option for participating in a national initiative is to develop a theme for a whole year in partnership with another ministry of your congregation. For example, the "Together We Can" program of Let's Move lends itself to year-round programming for children and families, and you may want to work with the Christian education leaders or the mission and outreach folks. There is a whole series of webinars for faith-based and neighborhood partnerships which address programs such as "Together We Can."

The options are myriad, but your choices should reflect the needs of your community and your team's interest in how to address them. There are certainly enough materials out there to keep your health ministry going for quite some time!

Accessibility

QUESTION

I'm concerned about accessibility in our parish. We have a wheelchair ramp, but how can we address other barriers that may exist?

There are good reasons to be concerned. As you probably know, the Americans with Disabilities Act (ADA) prohibits public accommodations, businesses, and transportation services from discriminating against persons with disabilities. Even though the ADA does not apply to religious congregations, making a church fully accessible is the right thing to do theologically and ethically. (Keep in mind the ADA may apply to nonreligious groups that use the facilities, such as the Boy Scouts or Alcoholics Anonymous.) A nice succinct legal analysis and summary of the ADA related to faith communities appears on the website of the Connecticut General Assembly.

In order to be accessible, a congregation will want to check the following:

- In addition to a ramp, do you have enough spaces designated for people who need accessible parking spaces?
- Once they are inside, can people get to the rest of the building, such as the fellowship hall or the choir room?
- Are there spaces for wheelchairs in the main sanctuary, or only at the back?
- Can people using wheelchairs get through the doors of the restrooms and reach the sinks and paper supplies?

There are other accessibility issues beyond mobility as well. Some of these include issues related to language. Many churches have found it helpful to have some (or all) of the following:

- Large print bulletins or lettering on the screens big enough to read easily.
- Bulletins in Braille for the blind.
- Assistive devices for people with moderate hearing loss.
- Interpreters who use American Sign Language for people who are deaf or profoundly hearing impaired.
- Language in at least part of the service that is accessible to children or people with developmental disabilities, along with use of visual aids such as art and music.

Repeating some elements (such as the Lord's Prayer, or the Doxology, or the hymn "Amazing Grace") also makes church accessible even to those for whom language is hard, including people with dementia. Often these familiar words and sounds remain long after almost all else is forgotten.

Then there are accessibility issues around feeling welcome in the church—barriers that can often be higher than any other:

- Are people whose sexual preferences differ from the traditional heterosexual preference welcome in the church?
- What about children with profound special needs?
- How about adults with mental illness?
- What about people living with HIV-AIDS?
- Are homeless people welcome?
- How would the church deal with a registered sex offender?

Other individuals may have personal barriers to full church participation that seem somewhat unique, but making a pastor, faith community nurse or health minister aware of the issue can lead to accommodations. For example, some people are highly allergic to perfumes or incense. Others with irritable bowel syndrome, celiac disease, or Crohn's disease may be reluctant to attend a church where there isn't a restroom in proximity to the sanctuary.

In my 20 years as a pastor, I have heard many reasons why people don't find the church accessible to them, but most of those reasons can be overcome with a little ingenuity and compassion. Just like the friends of the sick man, who lowered him down to Jesus through the roof of the house in which he was staying (Mark 2:4), we too, are able to find creative ways to open our sacred spaces to include all who want to be there.

Facing Pushback

QUESTION

We have a new pastor and now a member in the church is claiming that health ministry will cost more in liability insurance, but we have at least five times the cost of that insurance in the bank. What can we do?

Ouch! It has to hurt that you have been doing this work for years already and you have lost a true advocate in your former pastor. When there is a change in pastoral leadership, the bossiest people in church step up to the plate in the vacuum and start telling everybody else what they can and can't do. I'm wondering if your new pastor is in place. If so, run—don't walk—along with the folk you are including in your "we" above (because you aren't doing health ministries alone, are you?) and explain to the new pastor that the liability for health ministries is very small.

To clarify, if you are a faith community nurse, you should have a valid RN license, have completed a Foundations in Faith Community Nursing course, and be practicing your ministry under the Scope and Standards of Practice for Faith Community Nursing as developed by the Health Ministries Association and approved and published by the American Nurses Association. Your annual liability insurance would be around $200 or so from the Nurses Service Organization and the church would also have about the same expense for adding professional liability insurance for you. You should have your own, and they should cover you as well, despite the fact that the risk exposure is very small. Your denomination may have blanket coverage for health ministers. Check with your denominational offices for more information.

If you are not a health professional and you are doing health ministries, such as providing meals or visiting those who are homebound, your liability would already be covered by the church's policy that covers church volunteers.

The problem really comes with the scope of what you are doing. For faith community nurses, as mentioned earlier, the Scope and Standards of Practice are already clearly delineated, but there is no equivalent document for any other form of health ministry. You would of course not want to practice nursing or any other form of health care without a license and would operate under the Practice Act for your profession in the own state or province to reduce your liability risk (if you were, say, a CNA or LPN).

Get your health committee together and assemble your information about the scope of what you are doing, along with the cost and availability of liability insurance for your work (if needed). Then share that with your new pastor, the church trustees, and the administrative council. Actually, share this information with anyone who will listen. It might be a good idea to get on the agenda of the church's annual meeting if you can. Get health ministries added to the budget as a line item with a small amount to cover liability and a few materials (such as your bulletin board or printing materials to share with the congregation). Programs in the budget generally have more buy-in as they necessarily have more visibility.

Finally, document what you are doing (without sharing personal health information) and report to the church about what you are doing in the newsletter, on your bulletin board, through announcements, and through health promotion activities among groups in your church. Soon everyone will realize that health ministries are integral to any faith community called to preach, teach and heal.

Health Posters

QUESTION

My health ministry is currently limited to putting up a few posters around the church. In a year or two, I will have more time to offer, but is it even worth the effort to post signs? Do you have any data to support my efforts?

What you are doing is very important! You are providing health education, and we know that people often need to hear the same message multiple times in order to remember it. So keep on keeping on.

A recent study by researchers at Michigan State University ("Hand Washing Practices in a College Town Environment," *Journal of Environmental Health*, 2013, 75:8 by Borchgrevink et. al.) found that only 5.3 percent of people who washed their hands did so correctly, that is, washing with soap and

42   Health Ministry Advice for Everyone

water for at least 20 seconds. Most (about 90 percent of the women and about 85 percent of the men) washed their hands, but often without soap (22 percent) and almost always not for long enough. One interesting finding was that people were more likely to wash their hands if there were motion detection faucets, a clean sink, or a sign encouraging the practice. So, even just a sign can make a difference in hand-washing practices. And when the CDC tells us that there are 48 million illnesses in the US from contaminated food each year, half of which could have been prevented had people washed their hands correctly, that is a significant number!

Many public health campaigns are based on the fact that folks may not know some simple facts. For example, the "Know Stroke" campaign was based on the fact that only about one-third of adults knew the risk factors for and the warning signs of strokes (and what to do to if one was happening). Here are some important things to remember when posting signs or posters.

- Keep it simple. For example, if you are creating a poster about hand washing, you should include just basic information, such as the following: "48 million people get sick each year from eating contaminated food. Hand washing could have prevented half of those illnesses. Wash your hands with soap and water for 20 seconds." At the bottom, include the source of the information (in this case it was from the CDC), and a website where people can go for more information.
- Use pictures. This helps for the young and those who don't read English well. Use large print, and leave lots of white space. Again, the basic rule is to keep it simple.
- Change posters regularly. Once or twice a month is a good rule of thumb. Leave them up long enough to be seen, but not long enough to become ignored.
- Think "big picture" topics that will be of interest to many people, like a poster about the 211 Helpline where people can call for more information on a variety of services for all ages.

- Use reliable health information from sources such as the CDC, NIH, or well-regarded health organizations such as the American Heart Association or the Alzheimer's Association. Many good posters are available for free download on websites from reliable sources. For example, the We Can! program (Ways to Enhance Children's Health and Nutrition) has cute posters about children's activity and nutrition.
- Some of these organizations may also have campaigns you can support through a poster, such as the American Cancer Society's "Great American Smokeout," which is held the Thursday before Thanksgiving each November. With nearly 1 in 5 American adults still using tobacco, this is an important topic to highlight.
- Posters can be a way to solicit help for others, as well as a good message for faith communities to send. For example, the National Institutes of Health has posters encouraging people to consider enrolling their children in clinical research.
- Why not make some of your posters coloring posters and encourage kids to color a poster and take it home? The "Henry the Hand" site has some coloring book pages and posters about hand washing for kids.
- Try to match your posters to the National Health Observances. Several of the national health observances have free toolkits available, many with posters—certainly enough to have new posters every couple of weeks!
- Posters with sensitive information people might not want to be seen reading (such as about domestic violence or sexually transmitted diseases) could be posted inside toilet stalls. And you might consider having tear-offs on the bottom with a website or phone number.

Finally, make sure you put your health ministry name and your contact information on each poster. Ask the church administrator to print you out a few pages of labels with this information and stick one on each poster.

Health Concerns in Worship

QUESTION

I'd like to bring up health concerns in worship more often. Right now they just come up in our prayers and concerns. Do you know of any resources for this?

There are many ways to bring up health concerns in worship. One of the best ways is to include discussion of health issues in sermons. A Congregational Health Ministry Study done several years ago by the National Council of Churches found that when clergy preached about health issues, people responded, particularly related to health advocacy. The study found that "incorporation of whether or not the congregation heard sermons on health advocacy issues went hand in hand with an additional 17% increase of congregational advocacy by itself." For more information about this study, as well as sample sermons, visit the website of the Health Task Force of the NCC. Two collections of sermons and meditations that address this purpose are *I am the Lord Who Heals You: Reflections on Healing, Wholeness, and Restoration* compiled by Scott Morris, and *The Healing Word: Preaching and Teaching Health Ministry* by Deborah Patterson.

A second way to bring up health issues is by introducing programs that allow you to make announcements about health issues in church. For example, you might kick off a walking program by talking briefly about the high rates of hypertension or diabetes and the health benefits of exercise. Many congregational wellness programs are accompanied by information to share, and there are many reputable websites where you can go for more information.

Another way to bring up health issues in worship is to have a "Health Minute" as part of the announcement time. Also include a health blurb in your weekly church bulletin that is handed out prior to worship. Keep it short (a minute or two spoken, a paragraph written), but do this regularly, so that people expect to hear from you. These presentations can be done by the faith community nurse or by members of the health committee. You might want to also include similar items as part of weekly e-newsletters sent to members.

We are called to preach, teach, and heal, and all three should be organic to worship in every week!

Health Ministry Advice for Everyone   45

Health Ministry Sunday

QUESTION
Our health committee would like to plan themes for our health ministry over the coming year. Do you have any suggestions on how we could plan a year of programming in advance?

Any investment you make in planning will certainly help coordinate with other ministries in your church and will increase the impact you have on the health of the community. You might start by creating a year's worth of programming based on monthly national health observances. The National Health Information Center (NHIC) offers that information available online. Narrow your choice down to one a month, since there are several per month available. For example, April has eleven different health issues which designate that month as a focus, including Alcohol Awareness Month, National Autism Awareness Month, National Minority Health Month, and Sexual Assault Awareness and Prevention Month. Or, you may decide to set up a two-or three-year rotating schedule of monthly topics, similar to the Lectionary rotation.

From the NHIC website you can connect to a wide variety of national organizations, many of which will provide free health education materials to you. Most of them also maintain speakers bureaus and would be willing (with lead time) to provide a speaker to your group. For example, the American Cancer Society is often willing to provide a speaker who will come to your women's fellowship group to do a presentation on breast cancer.

Set up a bulletin board where you can highlight these topics using materials from these sources. You can find other health materials through your local county health department or local hospitals. Keep this bulletin board current. Put an article in your church newsletter (and your local newspaper), on the topic each month. Include a short blurb in your weekly church bulletin or in your weekly church e-mail. You might want to have a "health minute" announcement in church each week.

Work with the Christian education planners to see if your monthly health topic can fit in some way with what they are doing with both adults and kids. Or offer to provide one adult or children's education session per month on a health-related topic (again, relating it to the whole person as part of the faith community).

You may want to offer regular healing services. Abigail Rian Evans has a book called *Healing Liturgies for the Seasons of Life*, which has many good ideas for pulling together a healing service. There is much good music available, through Taizé, through the Iona Community (Wild Goose Publications), through GIA publications, and through the United Church of Canada (*More Voices* is their newest publication), along with many other denominational publications.

There is much that can be done. This is just the tip of the iceberg. But it is engaging work and can reap great benefits!

Finding an FCN

QUESTION
We would like to start a faith community nurse program in our congregation, but we don't have any registered nurses or much funding. Do you have any idea how we can start?

To be honest, it is unlikely you will be able to find a registered nurse who would be willing to volunteer a consistent number of hours each week in your congregation. But that doesn't mean you can't start a faith community nurse program! Here is what I suggest you do.

First, find out how much interest there is in forming a health ministry program in your congregation that includes the faith community. You might do this by taking a poll (you can find one in the appendix of *The Essential Parish Nurse: ABCs for Congregational Health Ministry*).

If you find that there is enough interest, then convene a meeting on the topic among interested congregational members. Discuss the idea and the results of your initial explorations. If you still perceive that there is interest in proceeding, at this time you will want to form a health committee, and brainstorm the names of about 25 individuals or families you might involve to be the founding sponsors.

At that point, ask each of these potential founding sponsors if they would be willing to donate two dollars per week to support the salary of a parish nurse. That would give you two hours of faith community nursing per week, and even two hours a week on a regular basis would allow for quite a bit of health education to happen!

If fifteen individuals or families each gave $10 per week, that would allow you to hire a faith community nurse for ten hours per week at $15 per hour, and now you are talking even greater possibilities.

Money to cover the cost of the liability insurance (about $150 a year), as well as mileage and other modest expenses, can be raised through one or two small fundraisers per year. This really is doable, so don't give up!

When you have the funding arranged, contact your local hospital and ask the Spiritual Care office for information about the faith community networks in your area. These groups can help you identify people who are looking to become faith community nurses. You will want to interview them, of course, if they are going to work for you. The person you choose will be employed by you, but he or she can participate in a larger network in your area. Networks exist in all 50 states and in close to three dozen countries. Depending on your denomination, you may have a faith community nurse network that can help you find a nurse that way, too. You will need to ask the RN if he or she has completed a Foundations in Faith Community Nursing course and holds a current nursing license. Once the person is hired, he or she should be encouraged to become active in a local network of faith community nurses.

Once you have hired a faith community nurse, he or she will need to get visible! Bulletin boards, newsletter articles, inserts in bulletins, and posters in the restrooms are easy ways for the program to be visible. Resources for these items are available in many places. Consider having the parish nurse share a "health minute" each week during announcements. Expect the parish nurse to participate in a documentation system, which is often available for a modest fee in a user-friendly confidential web-based program through parish nursing programs. This will help him or her to report (without divulging any private information) to the clergy, health committee, church council, or others who need to know this information.

Also, make sure the faith community nurse is included in your communications loop. All faith community leadership communications need to be well maintained to grow a healthy ministry.

Finally, make sure you celebrate the health ministry at least once a year with a "Healthy Taste" dinner. This is a great way to raise funds for the program, and to honor the supporters of the program.

Don't delay—start today! Faith community nursing can help share the load with clergy, and can multiply the ministries of a congregation.

Health Committee

QUESTION

It seems like having a health committee is more work than it is worth, as I end up doing most of the work as the health minister. Can you please give me one good reason why I should have a health committee?

Actually, I will give you 10 reasons, because if there is anything that a health minister needs, it is a health committee. But even more, your *congregation* needs a health committee. Here are my Top 10 reasons:

1. The church is called to preach, teach, and heal. Probably the church has a pastoral relations committee, or a worship planning committee, that supports preaching and worship. preaching moment. Your church also probably has a Christian education committee that undergirds the teachers, curricula, and educational programs. Your church also needs a health committee or health team to support the gospel call to heal (and much healing ministry is probably already happening).

2. Health ministry is a ministry of the congregation, not just of one person. You might have a wonderful choir director in your church, but without the choir, you won't really have much of a music ministry. The same is true for health ministry. The health committee is the "choir" for the work of healing in the church.

3. Having a committee working on a task creates buy-in for the implementation of a program. There is nothing worse than throwing a party and having nobody come. So throw open the doors and invite them to come in from the highways and the byways to the banquet of health ministry. It's a feast!

4. Many hands make light work. If you help people identify work that is meaningful to them, they will want to do it. Work together to help them select tasks that would give them purpose. For example, someone may love art and be willing to do a monthly bulletin board or posters. Someone else may love cooking and be willing to stock a few frozen meals in the church freezer for you to share with folks who need help during recovery from illness or surgery. Someone else may love to chat and be willing to drive someone to a doctor's appointment. You do health ministry because it is meaningful to you. Be sure that your committee has the same opportunity.

5. You don't have to meet every month. A health committee that meets quarterly can be just as effective (or more effective) than a health committee that meets monthly and gets burned out.

6. No one has to serve on the committee forever. Be sure to set up a plan for people to serve only for a year or two at a time, so that they can go off the committee without having to resign if their interests have changed. People are usually more willing to serve for shorter stints than for years on end.

7. When the pastoral leadership changes, you will want stakeholders in the congregation to understand the importance of this ministry and why it needs to continue. This is a very important reason.

8. Having a committee gives more visibility to a program that can often be invisible due to the private nature of many health concerns. You may be working very hard, but no one else may know it. Make sure your health committee knows it, along with the pastoral leaders, and the congregation's governing board. Document and share the aggregate data (not any private health information).

9. Committee members (not you) can suggest to the congregation that they need to pay a faith community nurse, or to set up a memorial fund where gifts can be given to support health ministry initiatives. And when there is a budget line item, there is additional visibility for the program.

10. It's a lot more fun to play on a team than it is to play alone. Jesus chose 12 disciples, not just one, so that they would work together, and he sent them out two by two. Health ministry can be hard work, and you need others to travel the road with you.

So go ahead, and choose five to seven folks of different ages, genders, and vocational backgrounds, and start meeting quarterly. Equip the saints to do this work with you, and this ministry will be blessed!

CHAPTER 3

Promote Wellness

Exercise Program

QUESTION
We are thinking of starting an exercise or wellness program in our church. Do you have any suggestions of how we could start?

Walking is the easiest way to include people in a wellness program, and data also shows that using a pedometer will motivate people to walk more. So will checking in with a buddy, someone you can visit with and keep you going. You can count steps—about 2,000 per mile—or you can track time—about 20 minutes per mile. And if folks are doing other exercise, such as armchair exercises, 20 minutes could count as a mile.

One popular program used by many congregations has been *Walk to Jerusalem*, often used at Lent, or *Walk to Bethlehem* for Advent. This program, written by Nancy Evans, is produced by St. John Providence Health System in Warren, Michigan. You simply calculate the miles between your congregation and Jerusalem or Bethlehem, and invite people to keep track of their daily walking distance and tally the total for the congregation each week. And you can grow it from there.

Nancy Evans also wrote the congregational wellness program, *Challenge Yourself, Change the World,* which connects wellness with social action and is a nice next step to follow the Walk to Jerusalem in the spring or in the early fall. You might also consider *Get My People Going!* (an eight-week intergenerational wellness program) available from the Church Health Center. The Church Health Center also has a superb year-long walking program, with Bible study included, called *Walk and Talk*. Be sure to check it out. And there are others—or create your own!

Finally, be sure to include spiritual support for your congregation's efforts with e-mails, bulletin inserts, or short newsletter articles. Here's an example:

Tired of exercising? Join the club! You are surrounded by a "cloud of witnesses" who would call you to "run the race with perseverance," so that we do not "grow weary" and "lose heart." (Read Hebrews 10:23–25 and Hebrews 12:1–2.) It's good for your energy levels, your spirit, and your heart to get up and move, so press on, dear saints of God!

Walking Program

QUESTION

We are going to be offering a Walk to Jerusalem program this spring, and we were wondering if you could give us some ideas on how to keep the program interesting through the weeks to keep people involved?

Here are a few ideas on how to support a walking program in your church.

- Good quality pedometers are really important. Research shows that people walk further when they use a pedometer—it becomes its own reward. You can ask people to buy them, or find money to have them donated for your program. The Community Church in Josephberg, Alberta, got a small government grant to cover the purchase of pedometers.

- The pastor's visible and ongoing support will mean more than anything to the success of this endeavor! You might want to have an announcement the first week in church to be sure that everyone knows how to use the pedometers and how to track their miles, with the pastor being the first to receive a pedometer.

- You might want to put a map up on the wall somewhere in the church where you can track the miles as they add up. Each week add a push pin and a slip of paper showing the date as a visual reminder of progress.

- Place blank slips of paper in a bowl at the back of the church and ask people to write their miles down each week. Ask them to put the slips in the offering plate and designate someone to add them up while others count the money. Those who might miss church for a week can e-mail the church secretary with a weekly tally. (And remember, 20 minutes of any mild exercise, such as gardening, or cleaning the house, can count for a mile.)

- Hang up pictures around the church of various places along the way to "see the sites." You can add the photos as you "arrive" at each place each week. Of course the European countries are the most varied. You will have to use your imagination when you are crossing an ocean.

- You might want to have a different person each week talk about why he or she is taking part in the program—to improve health, to get out and enjoy the fresh air, to have a chance to visit with someone they are walking with, and so on. This makes it visible that a number of people are involved.

- If you include music, that's another inspiration to folks to hang in there. For example, your church musicians might play the theme from "Chariots of Fire" while people are walking up to the front to talk about why they are participating. Challenge your church musicians to find other moving themes for each week.

- For snacks after church each Sunday, serve something from each area where you have walked. For instance, if you walked the distance from Alberta to Quebec by a particular Sunday, you might serve small servings of poutine (with gluten-free gravy).

- Send out an encouraging e-mail with a Scripture verse each week to everyone in the church.

- For the last week, you might want to have a "Middle-Eastern potluck" to have folks celebrating their success in walking to Jerusalem.

- Make sure you take pictures of the walkers (perhaps at the Middle Eastern potluck with their running shoes on). Local newspapers often are interested in covering stories about people working together to make positive changes in their lives and will appreciate your photos. Or take a picture of your group walking together when you start the program and send it to the paper to help a reporter who wants to track your progress.

Health Ministry Advice for Everyone

Clergy Health

QUESTION

My pastor is so unhealthy. I think it sets a bad example, but I'm uncertain of how to approach him. Do I have any right or is it even appropriate to do this?

If your pastor is unhealthy, he or she has plenty of company among other clergy leadership in this country! Documentation collected at Duke Divinity School as part of their Sustaining Pastoral Excellence Program shows that the most critical areas facing clergy were in the areas of "weight, mental health, heart disease and stress." This included information on the following studies:

- A national survey of more than 2,500 religious leaders conducted last year by Pulpit and Pew, a research project on pastoral leadership based at Duke Divinity School, found that 76 percent of clergy were either overweight or obese, compared to 61 percent of the general population.

- The same study also found that 10 percent of those surveyed reported being depressed—about the same as the general population—while 40 percent said they were depressed at times, or worn out "some or most of the time."

- A survey of Lutheran ministers found that 68 percent were overweight or obese, while 16 percent of male pastors and 24 percent of female pastors complained of problems with depression.

Source: FaithandLeadership.com

Several denominations have been concerned enough about this issue to create programs to help. For example, Gwen Halaas, MD, is the project director of the Ministerial Health and Wellness Program, an initiative of the Evangelical Lutheran Church in America to improve the health of Lutheran pastors and other church leaders. The Missouri Synod Lutheran Church helps to support the work of John Eckrich, MD, director of Grace Place Lutheran Retreats, which seeks to address the holistic health concerns of clergy and their spouses. The United Methodist Church has a number of outstanding programs to support clergy health and has issued a series of five recommendations to support clergy health.

One way to address this issue might be to plan a health screening program for your congregation and ask if the pastor would be willing to model support for the program by being screened. For example, schedule a mini health fair at your congregation, and arrange for local providers to offer a range of screenings. This might include hypertension, cholesterol, vision, hearing, bone density, and depression.

Congregations can roll out programs and the planning team can ask the pastor to show support by taking part in the program. Or they can offer "Healthy Tastes" at coffee hours or fellowship meals and ask the pastor to encourage people to take advantage of these healthy foods and make them part of their lifestyle.

No matter what your role in the congregation, it is always appropriate to say to your pastor that you are worried about the workload he or she is carrying, as well as the hours the pastor keeps and the impact this may have on health. That may open the door to conversations around other aspects of your pastor's health.

A less direct route would be to ask a church leader to contact the pastor's supervisor—if he or she has one—such as a bishop, conference minister, or district superintendent to ask the supervisor to address the issue. If you want to be sure you know what is said, however, and how it is said, it is generally better to have this conversation yourself.

It becomes even trickier when a pastor is leading a lifestyle that includes substance abuse. In this circumstance, going through the channels of church hierarchy is the best way to deal with the problem. Many programs help clergy and other professionals to deal with these issues, and the pastor's church-related health insurance plan could cover the cost. The pastor will need the support of leaders in the wider church.

Whatever you do, when you raise the issue of healthy lifestyle out of a genuine sense of concern for the well-being of your pastor, he or she most likely will understand that you are doing so out of personal care, not out of judgment.

Health Ministry Advice for Everyone   59

Healthy Meetings

QUESTION
Do you have any ideas for fun ways to incorporate wellness into committee meetings such as church council or Christian education committee?

It's great that you are aiming to include healing and wholeness in all parts of your congregation's work. Here are ten ideas for brief activities you might do within committee meetings:

- Create a timed agenda for your meetings, with each item assigned a start and end time. Keep your meetings to less than two hours. Schedule a ten-minute break halfway through to stand and stretch. Encourage members to get a drink of nice cool ice water or a warming cup of hot herbal tea.

- Build into the agenda a short video that will give you some good ideas about health ministry. One suggestion is the ten-minute DVD available through the Church Health Center called "A Look at Parish Nursing." Another might be the great video on exercise by Dr. Mike Evans called, "23½ Hours: What is the Single Best Thing We can Do for Our Health?" which teaches the value of exercise in a way that makes everyone want to run out the door. Perhaps it is best to show that at the end of the meeting!

- Take time for sharing a health minute. You can find many great ideas in Dr. Scott Morris's publications, *40 Days to Better Living* that focus on various aspects of health, from depression to hypertension to optimal health. Dr. Morris also has YouTube videos you might share.

- Have a five-minute "instant recess" when everyone is invited to get up for a minute and "jump around." This works well if you have some lively music ready to go.

- Invite people to bring a "Surprise Healthy Treat" to share with the group in the middle of the meeting, along with recipes for the new snack or dish.

- Take five minutes to tell the story of a health minister from history who made a real difference in the world, like Dr. Granger Westberg, who started parish nursing, or Quaker minister Elizabeth Fry, who was a reformer of prisons in Europe. Other international ideas include the people who started the Neighborhood Houses, the Salvation Army, the YMCA, or Deaconess movements. Or tell a story of someone in your community who founded a hospital or nonprofit organization.

- Enjoy a five-minute wiggle. Use one minute for your feet and toes, a minute for your fingers and hands, a minute for your whole legs, a minute for your whole arms, and a minute for your head and torso.

- Plan for five minutes of silent prayer and rest for renewal. It is well documented that meditation can have a very positive influence on health conditions such as hypertension, and silent prayer should be part of every worshiping community.

- Do deep breathing for five minutes.

- Join the choir. This is one "committee" that gets a workout every time they get together. Singing is great for your health!

Church Gardens

QUESTION

I would like to start a church garden, but I really have no idea where to start. There's so much information out there. Do you have some good starting points?

Unless you want to do it all by yourself, you'd probably better start with a good committee. You will want everybody to get in at the ground level. (Pun intended!)

Your committee might include:

- Someone from your congregational governing body who will keep your garden connected with the mission of the church and can help you get permission to break ground.
- A cheerleader, a person who can get everybody excited about a project in your congregation
- People willing to donate plants, tools, and other resources.
- Three or four representatives from various groups—youth, women's fellowship, men's fellowship.
- Someone who knows a lot about gardening in your area.
- Members who like to dig in the dirt.
- Someone who is good at organizing these types of folks and seeing that people follow-through.

At your first meeting, think about the mission of your garden. Why do you want to do this? What will this garden be for? Is it to teach the young people in the church about nutrition? Is it to reach out to the neighborhood kids or adults? Is it to grow food to donate to the local food bank? Is it to reclaim and green up some of the area around your congregation? Is it to be a peaceful, green space in an urban core where people can relax and unwind? Is it to be a memorial garden with a columbarium?

Once you have a sense about what you want to accomplish, you can research some best practices from elsewhere. If you would like to start a community garden, the American Community Garden Association has a wealth of information on their website. They also have a great curriculum (modestly priced) which you can order for the committee to work through during the winter months to learn more about asset-based community development, community organizing, planning for communications, fundraising, and partnership-building, among other topics.

If your garden is to be a memorial garden with a columbarium, you will probably want to work with a designer such as Columbarium Planners, Inc. Others can be found in your local area. If your garden is to be a green space for the neighborhood, check with your city or county council to see if funds are available to help with this project. In any case, you will want to be aware of any regulations that may relate to your garden.

Before you begin, consider inviting a speaker to come from another church that has already done this, to share some of the "fruits of their labors" with you, too. Keep the congregation informed, invited, and involved every step of the way, and watch your garden grow!

Healthier Coffee Hour

QUESTION

I would like to make our coffee hour healthier. But there is great resistance to getting rid of the cookies and coffee. Do you have ideas on how to introduce healthier options?

You may be surprised to learn how much your coffee hour is already helping the people who attend your congregation. According to the World Health Organization, loneliness is a higher risk to health than smoking and as great a risk as obesity. Here's the great news: the church already knows how devastating loneliness is, and that's why there *is* a coffee hour! And this is why the church has many other opportunities for fellowship and connection, as well.

To make your coffee hour healthier, be sure to reach out to the newcomers among you and include them in your conversations. Do you have name tags for folks? Are there designated folks in the congregation who are especially gifted at hospitality and great at making connections and introductions? Include them in this part of your health ministry.

Now, about coffee. There's good news, and there's bad news. Surprisingly, the good news appears to outweigh the bad. Coffee drinkers, compared to nondrinkers, are less likely to have Type 2 diabetes, Parkinson's disease, and dementia, and have fewer cases of certain cancers, heart rhythm problems, and strokes (although coffee won't *prevent* any of these conditions). This is good news for the average American, who drinks 416 eight-ounce cups of coffee each year, including those who prefer decaffeinated coffee. The benefits are from the coffee itself, not the caffeine, according to most studies. The bad news about coffee is that regular coffee can raise blood pressure, as well as blood levels of the "fight or flight" chemical epinephrine (also called adrenaline). So be sure to include decaf coffee in your coffee hour.

Now for the cookies. Start by offering healthier cookies next to the current cookies, along with a large print handout comparing them for nutritional content. The Center for Science in the Public Interest, which has a strong interest in nutrition and nutritional labeling, provides a number of great articles about cookies that you can draw from to create interesting handouts. You can also find great basic information about food labeling at the Food and Drug Administration website. This FDA document would make a great starting point for an interesting adult education class or a women's or men's fellowship hour.

Of course, add fruit. Cut bagels or other low-fat breads into smaller pieces, and from time to time, offer "healthy tastings" in mini-portions, with recipes available to take home. Change takes time.

$15 Coffee Hour

QUESTION

I'd like to see our church offer healthier food for our coffee hours, but donuts are quick, easy and inexpensive to bring. Healthier foods take time to prepare and cost more. Do you have any suggestions?

I recently heard Peggy Noonan, MS, RD, CDE, from Mary Bridge Children's Hospital in Tacoma, Washington, speak to a group of faith community nurses about this topic at the "Today's Child" conference of Northwest Parish Nurse Ministries. She was describing how she integrates the 5-2-1-0 program (Google it to learn more!) within her home church and she had a wonderful perspective about healthy foods for coffee hours at churches.

Peggy said that she could provide an easy-to-prepare coffee hour for her mid-sized Presbyterian church for about $15 a week. Here are some of her suggestions:

- Don't take away the donuts or cookies. If folks want to bring them, just ask them to make them smaller, and then people can have just a little if they like. Substitute donut holes for donuts, make smaller cookies—just an inch across or so—and if you have bagels, cut them into pieces.

- Add popcorn in bowls. Popcorn is a cheap and wholegrain snack. Leave off the butter and salt. Use canola oil to pop the popcorn to give a little flavor.

- Serve "spa water" alongside your coffee and tea. "Spa water" is water with cut-up citrus fruits in it, like orange, lemon, or lime slices.

- Buy a pound of cheese, and cut it up to set out with a box of whole grain crackers.

- Eight to ten large pieces of fruit, cut up, will make a couple of nice fruit trays.

- Gather folks twice a year to talk about the coffee hour. Peggy provides a handout with suggested snacks sufficient for a coffee hour for the church at a cost of about $15. She asks 26 people (half a year's worth) to sign up for one week each (just one—no more). If folks don't want to be bothered shopping for the food, cutting it up, transporting it, and setting it up, Peggy asks them to donate $15 and she prepares the food for their week.

- Keep gathering and sharing ideas for the group to serve new things that look fun, such as having a "garden" of bananas on one plate, and a "garden" of pickles on another.

- Remember that positive messages are so much more likely to stick than negative ones. Add healthy foods rather than banning the not-so-healthy ones.

- Get the kids involved in creating a coffee hour from time to time. The youth of the church will have to be eating healthy on their own in a few years and can help plan and serve some coffee hours, too.

- Enjoy a treat now and then—there are no "bad" foods. Remember the *Go, Slow* and *Whoa* categories of food? *Go* foods are good to eat almost any time. *Slow* foods are good to eat a few times a week, but not all the time. *Whoa* foods are once-in-a-while foods.

The tricks to Peggy's strategy seem to be: involve others to help play or pay, think simple in quantity (popcorn, spa water, fruit), and have fun together.

Snack Ideas

QUESTION

I'm tired of serving carrots and celery sticks, and I'll bet everyone else is, too. Do you have ideas for snacks that are easy and fast to prepare for a group, inexpensive, look good, taste good, and are different?

I have to admit, I really dislike those veggie trays, even though I know they are "good for me," and generally make myself eat some of each boring little vegetable. Here are a few ideas to spice things up a little that make great use of a variety of vegetables and a few fruits. Multiply each recipe to accommodate the crowd you are serving.

Jicama spears with chili and lime. This is a good way to introduce folks to this vegetable. Cut a jicama into small strips (julienned). Juice two limes, and drizzle the juice over the jicama in a medium bowl. Refrigerate about 15 minutes. In another bowl, combine 1 tablespoon chili powder, ½ teaspoon of cayenne pepper, 1 teaspoon sea salt (or less). When it is time to serve the jicama, set it on a plate, and dust it with the spices. This recipe will serve 6.

Celery with cream cheese and bruschetta. Cut celery into sticks, put a little lowfat cream cheese in each piece, and top with a little prepared bruschetta. (I like Trader Joe's, and a jar goes a long way.)

Crisp spiced garbanzo beans (chickpeas). Heat 3 tablespoons of olive oil in large skillet over medium heat. Drain a 15-ounce can of garbanzo beans, and blot beans dry on paper towels. Add beans to oil and cook, shaking the skillet occasionally until chickpeas are brown and crisp, about 10 to 20 minutes. Make a spice mix with either 1 teaspoon pimentón (a Spanish paprika), cumin, curry powder (or a combination of the above to make 1 teaspoon), along with a freshly ground black pepper and a little salt if desired. Sprinkle the cooked beans with the spices and continue to cook, shaking the pan a bit more frequently, until the spices are toasted and fragrant, 2 to 3 more minutes. Taste for seasoning, drain on paper towels if necessary. Serve warm or at room temperature.

Spiced melon balls. Use a melon baller to remove the flesh from a ripe cantaloupe and a ripe honeydew. Combine the balls in a bowl with these seasonings: 1 teaspoon ground coriander, ½ teaspoon cayenne, 1 tablespoon finely minced cilantro leaves, and 2 tablespoons freshly squeezed lime juice. Cover and refrigerate for up to 2 hours before serving.

Minced vegetable dip. Mince the following vegetables (or substitute others you have on hand): 1 cucumber, 1 red bell pepper, and 1 scallion. Mix them together with 1 tablespoon freshly minced dill leaves (or 1 teaspoon dried dill), along with 1 cup sour cream or plain yogurt. Add pepper (salt only if necessary), and a little lemon juice to taste.

Herbed cottage cheese. In a large mixing bowl, mix together 1½ cups nonfat cottage cheese and ⅓ cup plain lowfat yogurt, 3 green onions (chopped), 2 small garlic cloves minced, ½ teaspoon dry mustard, ½ teaspoon Worcestershire sauce, ¼ cup chopped fresh parsley, and 1–2 tablespoons of lemon juice. Pepper to taste. If you like, add fresh dill (¼ cup) or 2–4 tablespoons of chopped fresh basil, if available.

Navel oranges tossed in salsa. Cut oranges (heirloom oranges taste awesome in this recipe) in small bite-sized pieces and tossed with a non-sugary tomato-based salsa, such as "Pico de Gallo." You can find this salsa in a large container at Costco for a few dollars.

Baba ghannouj. Cut off ends of 1 large eggplant and bake at 350 degrees for 20–30 minutes until soft and partly collapsed. Peel and mash. (Or don't peel; the peel is edible). Mix together ⅓ cup lemon juice, with 2–3 minced garlic clove, 2–4 tablespoons of water, and 6 tablespoons of tahini until smooth. Add eggplant and continue mixing, adding liquid as needed. Chill for at least 3 hours. Top with a dash of paprika and serve with raw veggies or crackers.

Italian popcorn. For each eight cups of popped corn (popped in a heart-healthy oil), add 1 tablespoon of dried Italian spices, such as basil, oregano, or parsley, and a little black pepper. Pour the spices over the hot popcorn in a paper bag and shake.

Serve up each of these recipes with a generous helping of fellowship and fun!

Healthy Holidays

QUESTION

The holiday season is often an unhealthy time for eating, drinking, and exercising. What can we do in the church to encourage folks to stick with their healthy lifestyles?

As the church year begins with Advent, you might encourage folks to begin their New Year's Resolutions during this time, which will give them a jump on the calendar's new year in January. Remind them that healthy lifestyles are about adding good things to your life, like the glow you feel from a good workout, and not taking things away from them (like lying in an inert state on the couch or eating a warm sugar donut).

Why not build on the theme of the wise men bringing gifts to Jesus and encourage people to give themselves gifts of health during the Advent season? Here are ten suggestions for gifts from among which wise people might choose three for themselves to stay healthy during the holiday season.

- Take time for self-care with a massage, which helps promote the movement of fluids in the body through the lymph system, and releases stress from muscles and other tissue.
- Buy yourself a nice drinking glass to encourage yourself to drink more water every day.
- Buy yourself a new pillow and go to bed 10 minutes earlier than usual.
- Join a health club now and learn to use the fitness machines before the crowd gets there in January.
- Start an Advent walking group to walk through the malls and enjoy the holiday music.
- Laughter is a wonderful medicine, and the analgesic (pain reducing) quality of laughter is magnified when we laugh together. Go out with friends to watch a fun holiday movie together.
- Buy your holiday gifts at small local stores and avoid the stress of the big-box stores.
- Turn off the television—each hour you watch takes 21 minutes off your life. Watch a holiday movie on TV while you are doing something else, such as standing up and wrapping presents or doing some early holiday cooking to stick in the freezer.
- Mix up healthy holiday drinks, like sparkling water mixed with a little cranberry juice. Or try this healthy holiday nog: four bananas, 1½ cups skim or soy milk, 1½ cups plain nonfat yogurt and ¼ teaspoon rum extract. Puree all ingredients until smooth. Top with a dash of nutmeg.
- It is more blessed to give than to receive: get out there and help some other folks—at the food pantry, doing some home repairs, running errands for others.

Spiritual Health

QUESTION
If spiritual health is part of holistic health, what should I be doing to improve my spiritual health?

Here are 10 ways to improve your spiritual health as part of your physical health.

1. Take time to pray. If you keep prayer in your mind and your heart, you can pray at all times and places. But also take time to sit still and pray. Much data has related meditative practices to improved physical health, particularly around hypertension. Prayer can also help you clear your mind and find new vision for your day and your life.

2. Find a house of worship where you connect spiritually with the liturgy or music. Find a place where you also feel comfortable with the people you meet there. Attend worship regularly and sing along with those spiritual songs! Singing is so good for your soul.

3. Make friends with the folks you meet at church and find other friends who also will help feed your spirit.

4. Go for a walk every day, even when you don't feel like it and the outside doesn't seem very inviting. You will see the beauty in God's creation even on the stormy days, and your spirit will lift. If it is unsafe for you to go outside because of severe weather or a current health condition, take an eight-minute prayer journey around your house, and give thanks for the blessings you find—food, water, the roof, a warm bed, clothes, shoes, a memento from a friend.

5. "Blessed are the peacemakers" (Matthew 5:9). Work to make the world a better, safer, more peaceful place. Social justice was a big part of Jesus' healing message, and working for justice will bless your soul.

6. In the early church, feeding the hungry was an important task of ministry. Those chosen to serve in this way were called "diaconal ministers" (deacons and deaconesses). Feeding the hungry today will feed your spirit. Try volunteering at a food pantry. Buy some extra food each week at the grocery store to share.

7. Jesus said, "I am living water." Make it a spiritual discipline to drink several glasses of water each day, remembering that it is helping to cleanse and restore your body, which houses your spirit.

8. Biblical texts are filled with healthy foods, like lentils, honey, and herbs. As you read the Bible, watch for the way that food is described as part of a healthy life. What else in the Bible points to a healthy body and spirit?

9. Take time to dream. You need seven to eight hours of sleep every night. The Bible has a number of stories where God spoke through dreams, including Joseph in Egypt, and Jesus' father Joseph (who was told to flee with Mary and Jesus to Egypt). The prophet Joel talks about the Spirit of God being poured out and old men dreaming dreams (Joel 2:28). Be sure you stop at the end of each day and get a good night's sleep. You never know what your dreams might be telling you if you don't get enough sleep to pay attention to your dreams.

10. Every night, when you lie down to sleep, say a prayer to end the day. Here's a different prayer you might consider:

    Now I lay me down to sleep, I pray Thee, Lord, the world to keep.
    Grant peace-filled dreams, and guide my soul. Oh, keep my mind and body whole!

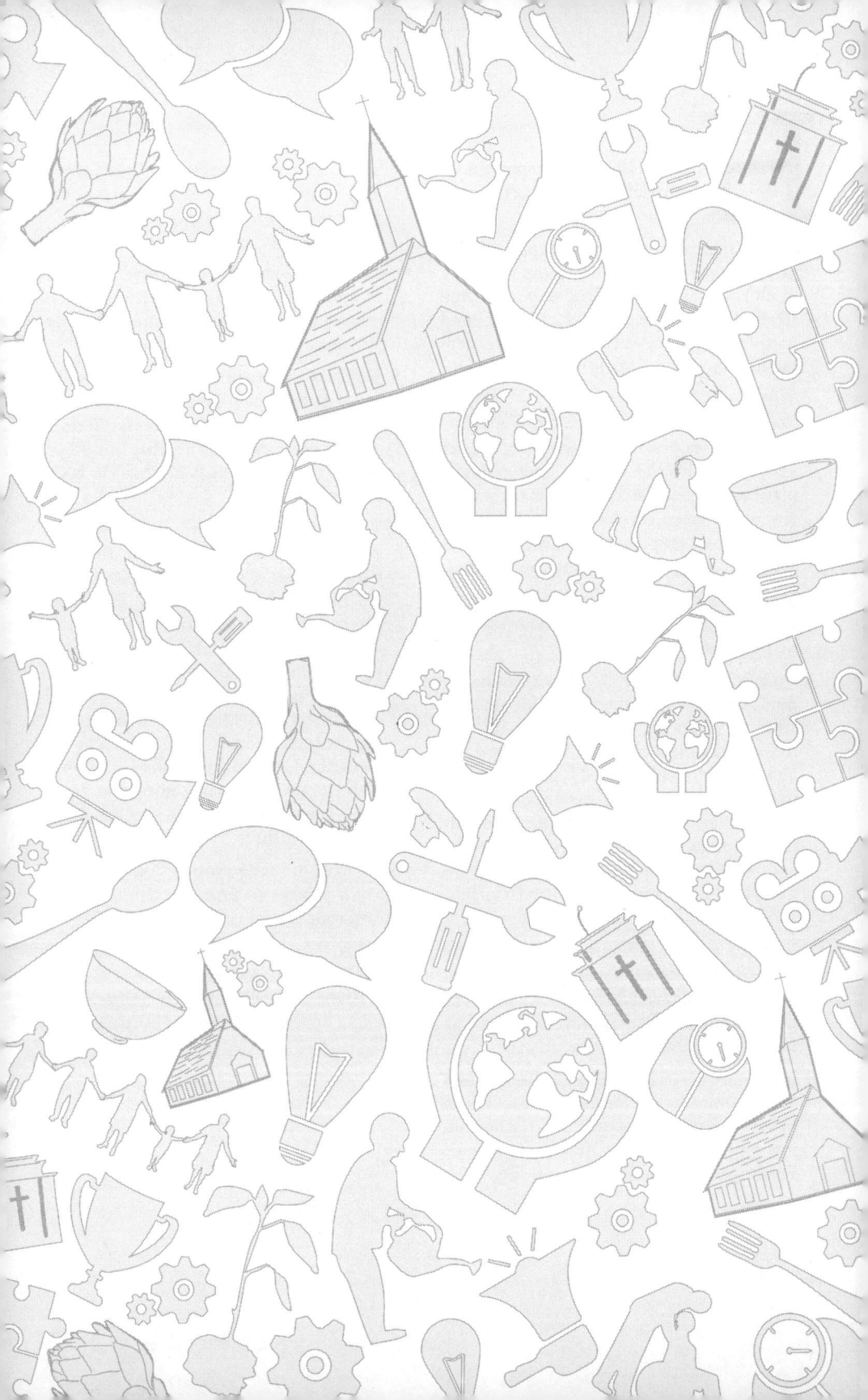

CHAPTER 4

Children, Youth, and Families

Children's Health

QUESTION

We would like to have an impact on children's health but we don't have any health professionals in our congregation. What can we do?

Here are some simple ways you can have an impact on the health of children.

- Preach it! If the pastor says something, it is more likely to be heard. Learn the statistics about children's health and connect this message with the theology of your church to tell folks why this is something that the church needs to be caring about. If you don't believe it, why should they?

- Teach it! There are so many free tools available online for health education, particularly around nutrition. The website ChooseMyPlate.gov has posters and coloring pages and other materials that can be copied for kids. And the Church Health Center's *Alphabet Appetite* is a great, affordable curriculum to use to support families' efforts to help their kids eat well.

- Allow it! We are always telling our kids not to run. How about creating a nice, safe spot in the church building or yard where kids can run around during coffee hour? This could even be opened up during the week for after school.

- Disavow it! If we stop serving donuts at coffee hour and serve grapes and cut up oranges instead, the kids will eat those.

- Show it! Let kids see you washing your hands or using hand sanitizer before you go to coffee hour. Let them see you taking the stairs two at a time. Let them see you playing an active game. Let them see you trying new foods.

- Grow it! Plant a community garden next to the church and include the kids every step of the way from planning to planting, from tending to harvesting, to cooking and feasting.

- Inspire! There are amazing people in your congregation who are inspiring and who can motivate kids to change their lives. Recruit them to get involved with this initiative.

- Perspire! Cardiovascular exercise is good for your body, burns fat tissue, and it's good for your brain. Try *Walk and Talk* (published by the Church Health Center) for adults, and have a *Walk and Talk* class with adapted discussion questions for kids at the same time.

- Test it! Call your local hospital or public health department to inquire how to arrange for free health screenings for your congregation. Don't give up until you find someone willing to provide screenings for vision, hearing, weight, BMI, and blood pressure.

- Best it! Arrange for the screenings to be redone a year later, and families can see if your efforts have paid off.

This is only the tip of the iceberg (but the bottom of the barrel for my rhymes). There are countless ways congregations can help improve the health of the children of the community, but it takes a village!

Childhood Obesity

QUESTION
We would like to find ways to participate in initiatives to address children's obesity. Can you give us any ideas on how we might get started?

Now is a great time to get involved! First of all, check out the "Let's Move!" initiative that First Lady Michelle Obama launched in 2010. There you will find data that supports the importance of your work: over the past 30 years, childhood obesity rates in America have tripled, with one in three children being overweight or obese. This dramatic rise is due to larger portion sizes, more snacks, and more sedentary lifestyles, including staying indoors and riding in cars to activities.

According to the "Solving the Problem of Childhood Obesity," a report by the White House Task Force on Childhood Obesity to the President, "one third of all children born in 2000 or later will suffer from diabetes at some point in their lives." The report also states that obesity can lead to chronic health problems such as heart disease, high blood pressure, cancer, and asthma.

So what can churches do? It turns out a congregation can do plenty! Here are some ideas to get you started:

- Plan an intergenerational walking program for your congregation. This sets a great example for kids.
- Include information about healthy portions as part of a healthy living curriculum within Sunday school or Vacation Church School settings. The website ChooseMyPlate.gov has materials that can be downloaded for kids, including coloring pages, posters, and games.
- Plan a screening for kids that includes a number of health screenings, such as vision and dental, so that weight and BMI screening are not the focus. Don't forget to screen for hypertension, which is growing among kids. You may wish to arrange for diabetes screening as well. Work with your local hospital to arrange this.
- Pull together a program that encourage kids to get out in nature during the week and connects them with the world again. The No Child Left Inside movement is a good resource.
- Visit local schools and see what's on the menu. Are there soda and snack machines there? Does the school partner with local farmers to get fresh, healthy food to serve the children?
- Start a community garden in your congregation and get the kids involved. Teach kids how to cook by using some of the food from the garden. Or arrange to host a Farmer's Market on your church grounds.
- Partner with a local community college to offer some cooking classes to the youth group at your church.
- Invite a local dietician to write a column in your church newsletter.
- Host a summer meal program for kids at your church with the help of the USDA. Information is available online.

Teen Obesity

QUESTION

I am worried about a number of teen girls in our congregation who seem to be overweight. Do you have any suggestions about how we can help them?

Are a number of the middle-aged and older women in your congregation overweight as well? (I'm guessing they may be.) What are the women of your community modeling as appropriate behavior for an adult female? Do they see you walking or biking around town? Do you have social activities at church that involve physical activities like hikes or softball in which women are equally represented? Do you encourage your parishioners to come to all-church picnics in the park or to all-church camps?

Second, what food is the church serving at various functions? A lot has been written about this elsewhere. For starters, see the answers on the $15.00 coffee hour (page 66). And for working with younger children to help them develop good habits before they become teenagers, check out the Church Health Center's *Alphabet Appetite* resource.

Third, does worship in your setting involve movement? You might consider installing a labyrinth for meditative prayer. A lot of kids spend time going around these in church settings that have them. Start an intergenerational walk and pray program, for example.

Having said that, the primary place where teens spend most of their time is at school. Get involved in promoting healthy foods in your schools. Ask if you can serve on the wellness committee of your local school district, or find a volunteer who is passionate about this issue. Encourage the schools to set higher standards. While the USDA has new guidelines for the meals that can be served, the guidelines do not cover snacks. According to the Food Research and Action Center, 40 percent of school-aged kids buy at least one snack, such as candy, chips or soda, every day. Your local schools can set the bars higher. They should not fund programs through the sale of unhealthy foods to kids.

While talking with the schools, check to see if the schools have recess and physical education. According to data from the President's Council on Fitness, Sports and Nutrition, only 8 percent of elementary schools, 4 percent of middle schools, and 2 percent of high schools require daily physical education, and the rates for schools that build in time for recess are similarly far lower than they used to be. Encourage your community's schools to become involved in the "Let's Move! Active Schools" initiative. This program is free and encourages a variety of physical activity throughout the school years, including the teen years when girls are more likely than boys to drop out of physical activities.

Here are several other options you might consider within your congregation.

- Create a pool of mentors for the teen girls drawn from women in your congregation who are active and enthusiastic about it!

- Develop work-group projects (supervised by at least two adults) where the youth in the church do projects to serve or to raise money for specific youth group activities, such as a mission trip.

- Encourage all youth to take advantage of the scholarships that your church may already have in place for them to go to church camp each summer.

One final note: often obesity goes hand-in-hand with poverty. Helping folks to get access to healthy food year-round is important. You might want to consider a community garden, cooking classes, or offering a school-aged summer food program (for which there is funding through the USDA). This is not an easy issue, but it is an important, and a life-changing one.

Intergenerational Ministry

QUESTION

We want our church to get more involved in supporting the health of children, but we have a lot more older people in our congregation than we have kids. Do you have any ideas about ways we could do this?

One of the beautiful things about a faith community is that it is intergenerational. And as Marilyn Johnson, faith community nursing coordinator in Vancouver, Washington, points out, those congregations that are truly intergenerational (that is, the different age groups worship together and do other church activities together) are far more able to keep their young people engaged in church when they are older than churches who send their kids away for children's programming during worship. So it is good for the health of the kids *and* the church when you do things together.

A good place to start for intergenerational health ideas is the "We Can!" program of the National Heart, Lung, and Blood Institute (NHLBI) of the National Institutes on Health. "We Can!" stands for "Ways to Enhance Children's Activity and Nutrition." Several different evidence-based curricula are available free on the NHLBI website. You will also find recipes, suggestions for activities, fact sheets, posters, tip sheets and more. Each family can call and order a single copy of the Parent's Handbook (1-800-866-35-WECAN), or that can be downloaded from the website as well. Free online training for leaders who will be using the curriculum is also available.

Here are quick ideas to get you started on intergenerational health programming:

- See if you can get a group rate for church members from a local swimming pool, or rent the pool for an all-church "Sea of Galilee Night."
- Plan an intergenerational softball or badminton game as part of an all-church picnic (to which folks are encouraged to bring healthy foods).
- Launch a walking program that invites people of all ages to walk and count their steps as they walk on an imaginary journey toward a goal that might be anywhere in the world. Places mentioned in the Bible, such as Jerusalem or Bethlehem, or locations where a church supports missions are favorite destinations.
- *Get My People Going!* available from the Church Health Center in Memphis, Tennessee, can be adapted for use by people of all ages. *Get My People Going!* invites people of all ages into a community experience of naming the areas where we need better health, and then making changes step-by-step that will improve health of body and spirit.
- Have the women's ministry plan and make healthy snacks for the kids at Vacation Bible School, and—very important—then sit down and eat them with the kids.
- Have the youth group plan and make a healthy meal for a "young at heart" group and have them sit down and eat with their elders.
- Plan a girls night out for girls and women of all ages with activities like Zumba, Tai Chi, yoga, manicures and pedicures and a healthy meal together.
- Have a movie night with a movie like "Supersize Me," which has messages about the stewardship of our earth and our bodies at all levels.
- Make healthy eating flyers for people of all ages—colorful, easy to read, with simple messages like, "Go, Slow, and Whoa! Foods."
- Some churches have "instant recess" where everyone who is able (at an appropriate spot in the service or coffee hour) stands up and moves to the beat. It helps to have an enthusiastic leader in the front getting everybody energized.

Online Safety for Teens

QUESTION

Our Christian education committee asked our health team if we would help them put together a program on helping to keep teens safe from online bullying and sexual predators. Can you help?

This is an important topic to address on behalf of today's children. The Internet has only been widely available for the last 15 years or so, so today's teens are the first generation to grow up awash in online and text communications. Most parents aren't as savvy as their kids in understanding these technologies and their uses. Here are some important factors to keep in mind as you begin to explore the possible impact of this technology on the lives of teens today.

- Many social networking websites allow kids to communicate with others online. Many of these have features that allow video chatting that may not be visible to parents checking a child's account.

- There are free programs (applications or "apps") on smart phones or tablet devices that allow a teen to anonymously "hook up" for meetings with people in their neighborhoods. These people may not have your child's best interest at heart.

- There are a variety of online chat rooms that attract kids around sexual topics. Teens find these at a time when they are exploring their sexual feelings and developing their identities. Again, the people they run into in these chat rooms are probably not the type of people you would choose as role models for your kids.

- Skype is a free online service that allows people to communicate by text or by transmission of video through cameras, which are in computers or easily purchased to use with a computer. It is a great service for communicating with family and friends far away without cost. However, this type of online interaction often gives a teen the illusion that one's communications are anonymous and safe, particularly if the teen does not give a real name or location. Teens often are lured to expose themselves under the misperception that this is safe and anonymous. This camera footage can then be captured as video and turned into pornography and shared with others.

- Photos of one's body taken by a cell phone can be forwarded to others or posted on social media.

- Unlike the threat of a predator lurking in the bushes, the online predator has the advantage of being able to form a trusting relationship with a young person over time before suggesting something further. Kids are so used to getting information online that often they aren't savvy about knowing what (and who) is trustworthy in the cyber environment.

- It is surprisingly easy for teens to hide such interactions from parents, given the easy access to communication through cell phone calls and texts, Skype, chat rooms, multiple free e-mail accounts and the like. Even iPods that are not cell phones have free downloadable apps that allow kids to text.

The fact of the matter is that online bullying and sexual exploration are widespread and growing, and the perpetrators are far smarter about the ways to lure kids and teens than most parents could possibly imagine. Do not offer a class to education parents about this topic on your own, but ask for expert help. Contact your local police department and ask for a recommendation of someone who can speak to this issue. I suspect you might want three classes—one for parents, one for teens, and one for pre-teens.

Do this sooner rather than later. Kudos to your congregation for not sticking their heads in the sand about this issue. You may be saving a child from serious and long-lasting harm, or worse. You owe it to the families in your church to help them navigate these relatively uncharted waters.

Advocating Public Policy

QUESTION

Our health team wants to address childhood obesity in a way that encourages systemic change. Can churches be engaged in public policy issues around health care without being too politcal?

While you cannot endorse a specific candidate for any election, you certainly can get involved with education about issues affecting the health and well-being of others, especially children who are depending on us. Addressing systemic change related to health practices is at least as important as encouraging individual change.

For the 16 million children (nearly 1 in 4) in America who live in poverty, healthy food and exercise programs at school may be their leading access to these important building blocks for healthy lives. According to Save the Children, 52 percent of children in rural America are overweight or obese. For 7.5 million children in America without health insurance, the school nurse may be an important link to screening and needed services.

If there are few healthy choices for school lunches, it will be hard to teach children to make healthy choices. If soda is sold to make extra money for the school, it is less likely kids will choose milk. Portion sizes are also 30 percent larger than they were forty years ago. Combined with the reduction in gym classes, the perception of safety issues related to outside play, the increase in screen time (computers, etc.), among other factors, it is no wonder that our country truly faces a childhood obesity epidemic with its related health problems, such as increasing rates of hypertension and Type 2 diabetes among kids.

So, how can you raise these issues? Here are a few ideas:

- Have a discussion within your health committee or adult education class about children's health issues. A speaker from your local hospital or a children's social service agency would likely be a good source of information to help jump-start the conversation.
- Educate yourself from other good sources. The US Department of Health and Human Services, in their *2008 Physical Activity Guidelines for Americans*, recommends that children and adolescents aged 6–17 have 60 minutes or more of moderate physical activity per day.
- Identify the most critical issue or issues you would like to address, such as junk food sales at schools, connecting schools with healthy local food, availability of time and resources for physical education and other physical activities, or access to health education and school nurse services.
- The church newsletter is a good place to share a summary of what you learned and what you believe should be changed for the good of the children. For example, you might consider writing an article about the "Farm to School" program, where local farmers sell vegetables and fruit to local schools.
- Schedule appointments to meet with school board members and principals to share your concerns.
- Encourage the parents in your congregation to be involved with the PTO and to raise these issues there.
- Write letters to those you are unable to meet with personally. Set up a table at church with information and materials available, so that parishioners can learn more and write letters raising the issue with policy-makers.
- Write to other local, state, and national policy-makers as well, sharing what you have learned and what you are recommending.
- Be sure that your own house of worship is acting on what is learned. For example, Save the Children has recommendations for healthy snacks developed by the Institute of Medicine and the Alliance for a Healthier Generation.
- The church can be a "moving place" in many ways. Plan ways to create church-related opportunities for physical activity for all ages!

Public policy is mostly about educating yourself as to what is happening and sharing what you have learned with those who have the ability to make positive changes. It is win-win for everyone!

Health Ministry Advice for Everyone

Domestic Violence

QUESTION
Our church would like to address the issue of domestic violence and childhood sexual abuse in our health ministry. Do you have any ideas on how to get started?

Intimate violence can take many forms. You are right to suggest that these are issues churches should be concerned with and raise awareness about. A number of churches are doing good work in this area, but that number needs to be far greater!

According to the Centers for Disease Control, on average, 24 people per minute are the victims of rape, physical violence, or stalking by an intimate partner in the United States. This comes from a 2011 National Intimate Partner and Sexual Violence Survey, or NISVS, a CDC public health surveillance tool.

On average, emergency rooms across the country see 84 children per hour for injuries sustained by violence. Not every injured child is taken to the emergency room, of course; many others suffer without help. State and local agencies receive more than six reports of child maltreatment every minute, and those are only the cases deemed serious enough for someone else to report on .

One clergywoman who has been working hard for decades to make a difference in this area, in partnership with congregations across the country, is Marie Fortune. A United Church of Christ clergywoman, Rev. Fortune has written a great deal about a faith-based response to sexual abuse and domestic violence. She is the founder of the Faith Trust Institute, which provides a wide variety of training and resources.

During one February, which is Teen Dating Violence Awareness Month, the institute hosted a free webinar on the topic of "Teen Dating Violence: What Parents Need to Know" presented by Rev. Al Miles. He is the author of *Ending Violence in Teen Dating Relationships* and *Ending Violence in Teen Dating Relationships: A Resource Guide for Parents and Pastors,* both published by Augsburg. The institute also has a wide variety of recorded seminars faith communities can use.

The Spiritual Alliance to Stop Intimate Violence (SAIV) is a program of the Center for Partnership Studies and was co-founded by author and peace activist Riane Eisler with Nobel Peace Laureate Betty Williams. Their goal is to help faith communities address all levels of intimate violence, including domestic violence, rape, child abuse, female infanticide, and other brutal practices. SAIV, whose advisory board includes folks like Archbishop Tutu, Harvey Cox, and Sister Joan Chittister, points to data showing that violent practices in the home and community make victims more prone to violent behavior, leading to greater violence in our society and in the world. Reading out to faith communities, SAIV says, "It is estimated that over 80 percent of the world's population belongs to a major religion. These people often look to their spiritual leaders for guidance. Yet religious leaders have been mostly silent on the issue of intimate violence. The greatest opportunity to reduce violence in the world is being missed. SAIV is working to change this."

What can be done? Start by learning all you can about this issue. The Centers for Disease Control, the Faith Trust Institute, and the Spiritual Alliance to Stop Intimate Violence are great places to start. They will have many ideas to help you educate the congregation. You will then have lots of ways to act.

Just-in-Case Bags

QUESTION

Have you had any experience with getting together little "just-in-case bags" for preteen girls who start their period at church? I think this might be something to have for the youth group leaders.

What a great idea! Here are some thoughts on this, and a tip received from Lisa Von Stamwitz, who served as Parish Nurse at Peace United Church of Christ in Webster Groves, Missouri.

Have the quilters or Women's fellowship (or health ministry team) sew up some small, fold-over bags out of nice upholstery type fabric, designed to be closed with a snap. Add a little button or bangle to make it look attractive.

In the bag, put the following items:

- Several maxi-pads—without wings, since they are easier for young girls to use
- Prepackaged wipes
- stain-remover pen

Those items address the immediate "feminine hygiene" need. But I would also encourage you to address a couple of other needs, as well. As congregations seek to address the wholeness of body, mind, and spirit, I would suggest you include three other items:

- A prayer bracelet with a red bead
- A red comb
- A red ribbon bookmark.

Include a page that says, "This prayer bracelet is to remind you that God, and your church family loves you. The comb is to remind you that you are beautiful, inside and out. And the bookmark is to remind you that your mind is beautiful, too. You are precious in body, mind, and spirit!"

Be sure you also include some basic health information that reassure girls that having their periods is normal and a wonderful part of life—a blessing, not a curse. Reassure them that they may experience some cramping and that they should ask a parent for pain medication. Remind the girls that they can ask their faith community nurse or a school nurse for more information or help.

You might also want to include on that same page a couple of links to good health care information for pre-teens and teens about menstruation, such as that found on the KidsHealth website (created by the Nemours Health Foundation) which has articles designed for different age groups (kids, teens, and parents).

You will want parents to know that you have these "just-in-case" bags for girls. The Mayo Clinic offers information for parents on preparing a preteen for her period.

Finally, talk to parents of girls with special needs to suggest that they have their daughters practice opening up, putting a pad in place, using it for a few hours, and properly disposing of it a few times once in awhile before they get their periods. That way when it starts they will be ready. It works!

Miscarriage

QUESTION

I think there are a number of women who have had miscarriages recently in my church. I'm unsure of what to do or how to approach them, if at all.

The best way to support those who have suffered a miscarriage is to open the conversation on the topic. The most nonthreatening way is to put an article in your congregation's newsletter, which should include facts such as:

- Miscarriage is the spontaneous loss of a pregnancy before 20 weeks, occurring in between 15–20 percent of all pregnancies (possibly more, since many occur so early that a woman might not have been aware she was pregnant). The language "spontaneous abortion" is not helpful. Stick with "spontaneous loss."
- Symptoms of a miscarriage and when to see a doctor (the Mayo Clinic has a good list, available online).
- Potential causes include genetic abnormalities or maternal health conditions, such as infections or uncontrolled diabetes.
- Risk factors, such as use of alcohol and nicotine, certain chronic health conditions, and age.
- What to expect following a miscarriage regarding your body and emotion.
- Self-care while considering another pregnancy.

Be sure to include your name, e-mail, and phone number, and ask people to call you with comments about the article. Remind readers that both your phone and e-mail address are private, so that any information they leave will be accessed by you alone. If or when they call, you can listen. Find out if a person would find it helpful to have a follow-up conversation, a referral for counseling, or the opportunity to be part of a conversation or support group with others who have experienced a similar loss.

You may also want to put up a poster in the women's restrooms simply titled, "Understanding Miscarriage." List the facts that you included in the newsletter article, and again, include your name, e-mail address, and phone number.

Be sensitive to triggers for people, such as Mother's Day, baptisms, the children's sermon, or the children's choir. Remember that everyone's situation is different, and people may be experiencing a range of feelings. The best things you can do are to provide information and an open door.

Holding Hope: Guidance for those Grieving Pregnancy Loss, a four-week Advent devotional, is a helpful resource for women and their families as they grief the loss of a pregnancy. The devotional is available from the Church Health Center.

Finally, here is a paragraph that you might want to include in a prayer on Mother's Day or other potentially sensitive times for folks who have lost pregnancies:

"Lord, we pray also for those who have lost pregnancies, that your loving arms would surround them in the womb of your Creation, which nurtures and heals all pain and sorrow. Bless and keep each member of your family in love and care. In your holy name we pray. Amen."

Adoption

QUESTION
Several families in our congregation are hoping to adopt children. Is there any way our congregation can help them?

Adoption is a wonderful route to a family, and it is one that is fraught with both joyous anticipation, and serious worry. It should be applauded as a wonderful choice, not a "second best" option, and fully supported by the congregation.

First of all, good information is key to a successful adoption. A number of churches have developed strong adoption support groups in their congregations. These groups provide education to those who are adopting all along the path to the creation of their new family configuration. Topics that should be discussed include information about the various types of adoption and what to expect along the way, such as international adoptions, domestic adoption of infants, and adoption from social service agencies within one's home state or another state. Additional sessions should cover topics such as attachment disorder, strengthening adoptive relationships, transracial and multicultural adoptions, foster care to adoption process, and post-adoption services. Most children who are adopted are considered typically developing, but in fairness to the child, this is not always the case. Some children experience neglect or trauma in their families of origin and face the adjustment of becoming part of another family. This can put them into the category of special needs, at least emotionally and psychologically. Like all children, adopted children will need plenty of tender loving care. Some will need additional counseling and developmental therapies, such as speech and occupational therapy.

Few people are experts in all areas of adoption, so here is where you will need to call upon expert resources in the community. You might invite parents who have already adopted, representatives from reputable adoption agencies with strong track records of support for adoptive families beyond placement, and representatives from the appropriate state social service agency that handles adoption. There are also wonderful groups of adoptive parents who may have speakers available, such as the Colorado Coalition of Adoptive Families (most states have one or more of these organizations), as well as special interest groups, such as Families for Russian and Ukrainian Adoption.

You might even get lucky enough to run across someone in your community like Melanie Sheetz, who is the amazing executive director of the Foster and Adoptive Care Coalition in Missouri (and an adoptive parent herself). Melanie and her staff put together a group of "extreme recruiters" who look for relatives who are willing and able to adopt children in foster care. Here is one of their success stories:

For three years, sisters Jada, Jasmine, and Jayla lived in three separate foster homes. They desperately wanted to live together. When Gayle Flavin, extreme recruiter, began this case, there were just six known relatives. Determined to find a forever family for these girls, Gayle and the extreme recruiter team got busy. Normally, it can take up to 24 months to find an adoptive family for a child, especially those considered hard-to-place: older youth, sibling groups, and youth with emotional, developmental, or behavioral concerns. The goal of extreme recruitment is to do this work in just 12–20 *weeks*!

Within weeks, Gayle found 146 relatives of these sisters! The next challenge was identifying the perfect forever family. Who of these relatives would have the space and the ability to care for these girls—together? The extreme recruitment team began reconnecting the girls with grandparents and cousins. Soon, a cousin was found who was eager to adopt the girls. "If I had known they were in foster care, I would have given them a home immediately! I'm so happy and know that the girls will be too!" After getting to know their cousin, the girls moved into their new home. Jada marvels at the resemblance between herself and a close cousin. Not only did she find a family with her two sisters, but she also has a new best friend.

Should this be a mission of the church? Just refer to James 1:27. "Religion that is pure and undefiled is this: to look after orphans and widows in their need." We do fairly well with the widows; what about the orphans?

Pregnancy

QUESTION

There are a lot of pregnancies in my parish right now. I think it would be fun to find a way to support these mothers-to-be. Do you have any ideas?

As a faith community nurse I knew in St. Louis ran a wonderful program for new moms-to-be for a number of years. Her program included regular group meetings in a quiet and comfortable parlor with cozy chairs where the women would gather for sharing health information and other support. (The meetings also included childcare for those who already had children.) In addition, she arranged with the pastor for a quiet time of prayer for the blessing of the pregnancies among the group. She was sensitive to the fact that this service of blessing would need to be a private time, just for those who were expecting, and for their spouses and any other family members or friends they wanted to invite. It was not held during the regular worship service for several reasons, most importantly in order to not add to the grief of any families who may have recently lost a pregnancy.

Many congregations offer Mothers' Day Out programs, but a nice alternative would be to offer a Moms-to-Be Night In, where pregnant women can gather together at the church in slippers and comfy lounging clothes to enjoy some healthy treats and beverages, and a movie or gentle dance music. Or they can just sit and talk together about their joys and concerns.

It might not hurt to invite an OB-GYN physician or nurse with great people skills to come talk with the group once every few months. For first-time moms, a little extra time in a supportive and nonthreatening environment with someone who has a depth of knowledge and experience might be comforting. The data show that group health education is often more effective and reinforcing than individual health information. What people learn in a group seems to stay with them longer, perhaps because they are less pressed for time, or the environment is more conducive to learning than a quick office visit.

Be available to answer questions. Make sure that the moms-to-be have your e-mail address and your cell phone number. They may want to ask you something personally that they would be afraid to ask in a group. You might want to have a standard book on pregnancy that you make available. Or you might want to have a small lending library, but I wouldn't count on getting the books back for awhile (if ever) after the babies are born!

Be sure to let the moms-to-be know that you will be there for them after they give birth, too. Postpartum depression is a real affliction for many new mothers, and you will want to be supportive. The church can be a great help in staying connected with and supporting new parents during such a tumultuous time. Some of the grandmothers in the congregation can be particularly helpful. Clergy and faith community nurses should be aware that postpartum depression may need treatment and refer the mom to her physician. Be sure to share this message with your new moms group, too.

Here is a prayer of blessing for mothers-to-be:

God of all mothers, we pray that you would be with [name(s)] as she [they] await the birth of their child [children]. As you blessed Elizabeth and Mary during their pregnancies with hope and joy, strengthen and support these women who await their precious ones. May their pregnancies be a time of preparation and renewal, and may the journey they have begun be one that has far more happiness and peace than worry and pain. Bless the children who are coming, and keep them safe in your loving care. Be with the families and friends who surround them all, and may their coming into this world be through your gentle hands. All this we pray in your precious and holy name. Amen.

Eating Disorders

QUESTION

I am worried about some girls in our church who seem like they aren't eating enough. For some families whose daughters (or sons) may have an eating disorder, this is extremely scary. Is there any way the church can help?

Eating disorders are scary, and families often think they need to hide them as a shameful secret. While the prevalence of eating disorders among the general population is relatively small (less than 5 percent of the population will develop an eating disorder over their lifetime), it can be very damaging to one's health, and sometimes life-threatening. According to the National Institutes of Mental Health, among females ages 15–24, the mortality rate from eating disorders is twelve times higher than the death rate due to all other causes of death.

Even if a person doesn't die from an eating disorder, eating patterns can lead to many health problems, including dry skin, severe constipation, anemia, infertility, low blood pressure, muscle weakness or wasting, osteopenia or osteoporosis, brain damage, and multiple organ failures.

It is time to talk about this issue in the church! And there is good information available. But it's tricky, because this is a hard thing to preach about. Where do you start to raise the issue among members of the congregation and to reach the families you are trying to reach?

First, some basic information: according to the National Institute on Mental Health (NIMH) there are three main types of eating disorders.

1. Anorexia nervosa—extremely restricted eating
2. Bulimia nervosa—binging followed by purging, excessive exercise, or fasting
3. Binge-eating disorder—losing control over the ability to stop eating

The NIMH has a detailed booklet that describes the symptoms and treatment for eating disorders available to download online or order in print from the NIMH.

Another great source of information is the National Eating Disorders Association (NEDA). They offer toolkits for parents, educators, and coaches, which are free to download online. They offer good information that you can use to create an article for your church newsletter, or for a bulletin board on the topic.

The NEDA website also has a toll-free number teens and families can call for help to locate treatment and support groups. It is 1-800-931-2237 and is available 9–5 Eastern Standard Time. You might want to create a small poster about this subject for the inside of a bathroom stall. These teens would be likely to use the restroom, and this would be a good place to put the toll-free number. NEDA also has an online screening tool, and information about research and other resources.

Having a regular, five-minute health session at each of the youth group meetings might be helpful. Then this topic could be covered as one of a series, rather than a big heavy topic at one gathering.

How else can you help? Check around to find out who treats people with eating disorders in your community. Invite someone to come and give a talk to the adult education group or the women's fellowship group. As a resource referral specialist, you are going to need to know where you might point people to get some help. People generally need counseling, medical treatment or both to deal with an eating disorder.

Remember, eating disorders are a leading cause of death. People with anorexia are 18 times more likely to die early than are peers of their age group. Our calling to preach, teach, and *heal can save lives.*

CHAPTER 5

Medical Issues, Education and Prevention

Prayers for Medical Procedures

QUESTION

A loved one recently fasted before a colonoscopy and I thought that medical fasting could be less scary if accompanied by some prayers. Do you have any prayers for fasting before medical procedures?

Fasting has a long and distinguished history in various religious traditions, from the daily fasting during Ramadan among Muslims, to the fasting of Jesus and others from the Judeo-Christian Scriptures. Being a little scared before a medical intervention, particularly one that involves vulnerable parts of ourselves, also has a long history. We give thanks for the blessing of safe and effective anesthesia!

Part of the preparation for a colonoscopy involves a jarring departure from our routine the day before—namely foregoing breakfast, lunch, and dinner. This day seems very long, indeed. There is also the additional worry about "What if they actually find something?" And "Well, if they do, I hope it's very small." And "I know somebody who died from colon cancer." We push away those nagging thoughts, but they are, frankly, what has brought one to do this.

Prayer on this day can take many forms, and I would invite you to consider a series of prayers that will help you through. You are being asked to drink a liquid that will require you to spend much more time than usual in a restroom. As one's body is being cleansed for the procedure, prayer can help retain one's composure and dignity.

Here is one possible series of prayers for this preparation day:

- **Morning.** A prayer of welcoming the new day. This day will be different than most. Ask God to help you be open to the new things you observe about yourself and the world around you as your routine is varied this day.
- **Mid morning.** A prayer for spiritual food. This might be a long day without meals, so pray that God would bless you with spiritual food this day.
- **Mid day.** Consider taking a short walk prayer walk around the block, or on a labyrinth. Or, if you prefer to stay near plumbing, find a finger-labyrinth online.
- **Mid afternoon.** A prayer of thanksgiving. Give thanks for the opportunity to have this procedure in order to take good care of your health.
- **Late afternoon.** Quiet prayer in a chapel or sanctuary setting. Absorb the peace that such a setting provides. Listen for that still, small voice of peace.
- **Early evening.** A singing prayer. Find a favorite hymn or spiritual song and quietly (or loudly) sing the words of comfort that will come to you again tomorrow. Or choose a favorite poem or Scripture to reflect on.
- **Before bed.** A prayer of release. You have been released from the preparations, and all you need to do tomorrow is show up. You are in the good hands of your doctor, and the even better hands of your God.

Remember: God gives sleep to the beloved (Psalm 127:2). And you will have even more sleep after the procedure is over. Relax. As Julian of Norwich said, "All will be well."

Surgery Support

QUESTION
How can faith community nurses and health ministry teams be helpful when members of our congregation are undergoing surgery?

- **Be sure the parishioner understands the surgery.** *A faith community nurse can ask if the parishioner has any questions* about the surgery, the health condition, or the expected recovery. Talking with a trusted health professional may help alleviate some fears the person faces. A faith community nurse can help identify questions need to be addressed with the surgeon.

- **Connect with the health care facility.** Ask the person undergoing surgery to *inform the health care facility* which church he or she is affiliated with and the name of the clergyperson or FCN, even if the facility does not ask.

- **Make sure the patient understands discharge instructions.** If the surgery is major or complicated, inquire of the patient whether you have *permission to talk with the case manager* in charge of discharge planning. The parishioner must give you permission to receive this information. It could be as simple as a form you create which says this: "I (NAME), give permission for my faith community nurse (NAME), to be informed about my discharge and treatment plan." (SIGNATURE).

- **Be present during discharge.** If the patient is cognitively disabled or elderly and alone, you might *offer to be with the patient during discharge*. One older parishioner had a pacemaker implanted, but didn't catch the discharge instruction to stop taking the medication she had needed before receiving the pacemaker. The parish nurse later checked on her, found her doing poorly, discovered the reason, and was able to intervene. Medically this person had no need for home health at discharge, so no other health professional would check on her. Again, you will want to have the individual sign a form similar to the one above, giving you authorization to be present.

- **Build a bridge back home.** Jeanne Brotherton, NPNM network coordinator with PeaceHealth in Bellingham, Washington, reminded me that many faith community nurses can assist with getting someone's *home ready for post-op time*. She says, "It's amazing how difficult it can be to do Activities of Daily Living (ADLs) when one can't walk well, can't sit well, gets dizzy with pain meds, and so on. Having ADL aids available, as our church does, or knowing where one can easily obtain items like a shower chair, a commode, specialized pillows, cane, or walker, is an important service. You can also offer to enlarge take-home instructions so they are easy to read. Make a list of items someone might think of having at their bedside (or in a tote that can be carried around) for the first few days—water mug with lid and straw, cell phone or cordless phone with phone list of numbers programmed, tissues, devotional material, remote control, meds or the daily schedule for those, and so on."

- **Include the whole health ministry team.** Inquire whether the person has *someone lined up to help them get to the surgery and home again*. Can a trusted friend stay with the patient overnight? Who will bring meals for a few days?

- **Connect back into the faith community.** Particularly if a person has undergone surgery for something like repair of a broken hip, there may be a fear of getting back out. Yet studies show that *getting back connected and busy again* is helpful both for discomfort and depression that may accompany isolation and pain. A member of the faith community can visit, pick up folks and bring them to church and to fellowship gatherings, and can get them reconnected to others.

Fall Prevention

QUESTION

Our church seems to have had an increase in falls lately—there are three people currently bedridden with injuries to their legs and backs. Is there any way we can help with fall prevention?

Kudos to you for asking the question, and not just assuming that everybody knows enough to avoid slippery throw rugs and electrical cords! There is a lot more to "balance" around fall prevention and recovery than first meets the eye, and a faith community is a great place to address the issue.

Here's why: research shows that after people fall, they are very scared about reinjuring themselves, or causing a new injury. And with good reason! Who would want to go through that kind of pain, and through that lengthy recovery period again? Along with the fall comes plenty of time for introspection and question asking. "What should I have done differently?" "Are my bones getting weak?" "Should I start to curtail my activities?"

Data show that up to half of older adults experience fear of falling (Howland, Peterson, Levin, Fried, Pordon, & Bak, 1993), and many therefore reduce their activities according to the National Council on Aging (Tinetti & Speechley, 1989). And according to A Matter of Balance, a program of The Roybal Center for Enhancement of Late-Life Function at Boston University, "being inactive results in loss of muscle strength and balance. It can also compromise social interaction and increase the risk for isolation, depression, and anxiety. Fear of falling can actually contribute to falling."

But there is help! A recent study at Boston University with SeniorMetrix found that when people broke their hips, attending a support group helped them overcome their fears of resuming normal activity. And where can you better find support than a congregation? Someone from the church can pick up the person at their home (making it easier to get from the house to church without having to find a parking space), and serving as a companion for emotional support—and a friendly arm—while walking.

Education is key. A majority of falls occur during routine activities, and many of those falls are preventable. Usually, falls are caused by more than one issue. Another important element of fall prevention is improving one's strength and balance.

There is a wonderful evidence-based program developed by MaineHealth called, "A Matter of Balance," which is led by a trained lay person who offers one or two two-hour sessions each week for eight weeks. The classes provide information about fall prevention, and simple strength and balance promotion exercises. This program is quite expensive—$1,500 to train one lay person, plus travel and lodging at the MaineHealth location. But if several churches shared the cost of training that person, or if you could locate a grant to cover the expense, it would be well worth it. Among those who have taken the eight-week class, 97 percent are more comfortable talking about fear of falling, 97 percent feel comfortable increasing activity, and 99 percent plan to continue exercising. Great news!

Or, ask a health professional in your community to educate folks about falls. Also, a qualified trainer could teach simple strength and balance exercises, such as Tai Chi.

Sleep Education

QUESTION
I'm worried that many parishioners aren't getting enough sleep. Do you have any suggestions for addressing this issue?

You are right to be concerned. According to a report from the Centers for Disease Control and Prevention, nearly a third of all working adults average six hours or fewer of sleep per night. This is a major public safety issue, as sleep deprived individuals are far more likely to be involved in accidents on the road, at home, or at work.

While putting together the "Keep Your Mind for Later Use" congregational brain wellness program for Northwest Parish Nurse Ministries, we learned that getting the right amount of sleep is a critically important protective factor for our brains at all ages, especially for middle-aged and older adults. A 2008 study funded through the National Institute on Aging found that folks who get less than seven hours of sleep per night have cognitive function equivalent to that of folks who are seven years older. Also, sleeping too much (more than nine hours per night) was hard on the brain. Seven to nine hours per night seemed to be the best for protecting cognitive functioning.

Here are ways you can address sleep.

- Invite an expert on brain health or sleep disorders to come and talk with folks at your church.
- Write an article on the topic for your church newsletter.
- Create a bulletin board with some facts about the topic.
- Ask the pastor to mention the issue in a sermon.
- Offer the "Keep Your Mind for Later Use" program in your church.
- Remind folks that cutting back on caffeine and alcohol consumption, reducing sugar intake, eating smaller meals, avoiding eating before bedtime, and getting some exercise every day are helpful with sleep.
- And remind them that, "God gives to his beloved sleep" (Psalm 127:2).

Funding an AED

QUESTION

We would like to get an AED for our congregation, but we know that they are quite expensive, and didn't know if there was funding available to help fund its purchase. Could you please help us?

There are a variety of ways to find local funding for an Automatic External Defibrillator (AED). You can get a portable AED, like most everything else, on Amazon.com or through Costco for about $1,200. But you might want to check with your local EMS office, fire department, American Red Cross office, or community education department at a local hospital for brands and sources they recommend. These community services also may be aware of grants available for the purchase of an AED in your area. Generally, an AED designed for use in a community setting would cost about two to three times as much as a home AED. You may also visit the websites of local or corporate foundations for grant guidelines. Some foundations, such as Medtronic's, have funded the purchase of AEDs since their use is closely aligned with the corporate mission.

Some health committees have simply asked congregation members if someone would be willing to donate funds to purchase an AED. That is how Ruth William's church, St. Mary's in Richland Center, Wisconsin, got one—from an individual donor. Other congregations have raised funds through bake sales or drawings.

The National Center for Early Defibrillation has a helpful step-by-step planning guide online to help you locate sufficient funding to acquire an AED for your organization. Their website states "that the first step is to estimate projected program costs.

Annual costs can include:

- Devices (about $3,000 per unit; remember to divide initial cost by the projected life of the device, usually five years)
- Peripheral equipment costs (about $75 per device)
- Maintenance (about $100 per device)
- Insurance (variable)
- Training costs (variable: includes personnel and equipment)
- Program management costs (variable)
- Event documentation costs (variable)
- Quality assurance tools (variable)
- Community-wide CPR training (variable)

They also point out that other sources of funding can include local corporations and industries, civic organizations, private foundations, public charities, and government grants.

After you have an AED in place, you will want to arrange for training. Most of the units are very user-friendly, but the training will give you much more information about use of the device with various age groups and situations. You can easily find training through the American Red Cross.

The appropriate church leadership body will want to decide who should be trained—the health committee, the ushers, the professional staff, or all of the above. The training can also be expanded to include First Aid.

Red Cross training meets OSHA guidelines and many other professional standards. They also offer continuing education units (for a fee), which may be helpful for health care professionals in many states. Again, you will need to decide who will pay for the training and how to raise those funds.

The bottom line is that you just might save a life. And every life is worth saving!

Health Ministry Advice for Everyone

Using an AED

QUESTION
We have an AED (automated external defibrillator) at our church, but don't know what to do if someone has a terminal illness and may not want to be resuscitated. What should we do?

Well, as Good Samaritans who tried to help, you probably would be forgiven by the person you helped—eventually! But as compassionate people of faith, you probably want to do the thing that causes the most beneficence, also known as the least harm.

First of all, your AED should only be used by those who are trained to use it, and these typically are members of the health committee and the ushers. In some states, such as Wisconsin and South Dakota, people who have a "Do Not Resuscitate" order, which they have discussed with their doctor, may have a special bracelet (called a "Comfort Care" bracelet in South Dakota) which states that they only want to be kept comfortable, but do not want any resuscitation attempts from health care professionals. Other states, such as Oregon and Washington, have a POLST document, which stands for "Physician Ordered Life-Sustaining Treatment." Again, this is information that would have been discussed between the patient and the physician. The bright red form on which this information is documented is generally kept in a visible place (such as the fridge door) in a person's home, but where would you find it at church, and does it apply to non-medical personnel?

According to Gretchen Brauer-Rieke, RN, MSN, certified advance care planning facilitator, the POLST form does *not* apply to non-medical personnel, and the person may or may not have a copy of the form with them to inform people of their wishes. It would be best if a faith community nurse talked with anyone known to have a terminal condition to inquire about advance directives and other forms such as a POLST and asked to keep a copy of the forms in a sealed envelope in the church office. In addition, the parishioner should have a sign (such as a Do Not Resuscitate designation on the back of their name tag) that the ushers would be trained to look for before using the AED. It would be the responsibility of the person to wear the agreed-upon "signal." Of course, in all cases where someone has collapsed, 911 should be called, and in the cases of states with a POLST registry, if the EMT has the person's name, they can often look them up en route to see if they have made known their wish not to be resuscitated.

Removing clothing to use the AED, breaking ribs through compressions of CPR and causing enough recovery to survive on a ventilator may absolutely be against the wishes of someone with a terminal illness. Education of church-based first responders should include information, along with a policy and procedure for compassionate care of people at all stages of life.

Blood Pressure

QUESTION

Every time anyone goes to the doctor, they get their blood pressure checked. They can also get it checked at the drug store and other places as well. Why should we bother with checking anyone's blood pressure at church?

I used to think that taking blood pressure was a poor use of a faith community nurse's time, for the same reason, along with the observation that there are always many other things that a nurse could be doing. Taking blood pressure measurements sure doesn't seem like capacity building. It would be so much greater to spend that time on developing a class on, say, cognitive well-being for middle-aged and older adults.

What changed my mind about regularly offering blood pressure readings as a critical part of a health ministry program was a little exercise we did at a monthly meeting of faith community nurses in St. Louis a few years ago. I have forgotten what the issue was that we were talking about that day, but as part of an exercise to get people talking to one another, I had them role-play the nurse-patient relationship. One nurse pretended to take the blood pressure reading of another nurse, and then they switched. What happened was jaw-dropping. In the course of less than a minute, those nurses who were "having their blood pressure taken" began to talk about health issues, along with things on their hearts. It was clearly an important entry point for beginning conversation about issues of body, mind, and spirit with people who were instantly perceived as trusted professionals.

Now the seasoned faith community nurse would know when to ask, "Would it be okay if I shared your concern with the pastor?" He or she would also know when to suggest a referral to a doctor, mental health professional, or other community resource. But having a regular time and regular place when a person can think, "You know, I'll just have my blood pressure taken," is great door-opener for those who might not think of "bothering" the faith community nurse at another time. And as long as the nurse is there, parishioners can ask a question or say what they have been worried about.

Having the regular opportunity available for folks to get their blood pressure checked helps to raise the visibility of a health ministry program. Folks may not need your services now, but seeing you and your team over and over will remind them that you are there.

It also seems to be helpful to request that everyone who is going to participate in a church-related wellness program have their blood pressure taken before starting. Some of those really healthy people may not have had their blood pressure checked for years, even decades, and you may help someone who is at high risk for stroke and doesn't know it.

One final note: offer to check the pastor's blood pressure once in awhile, too. And don't forget yourself!

Heart Disease

QUESTION

I know that heart disease is the leading cause of death in the United States. Is there any way that a congregation can help address this issue?

When I was in seminary, I was taught to preach both the scandal and the good news of the gospel—to be both prophetic and pastoral. So we need to hear and tell the figures like those shared by Louann Rondorf-Klym, RN, MS, a parish nurse in Wilsonville, Oregon, who presented on this topic at the Parish Nurse Network of Washington County, near Portland. She shared that one in four women die of cardiovascular disease, twice as many as are diagnosed with breast cancer (not that this is a competition, but the figure is startling). In addition, nearly two-thirds of women who died suddenly of coronary heart disease had *no* previous symptoms. One in four men also die of heart disease, although they usually have some symptoms more commonly associated in the public's eyes with heart disease.

What is the good news? We can do much to prevent heart disease—by keeping hypertension, weight, and cholesterol under control, for starters. We can do much to treat heart disease. The support of a faith community can make all the difference in the world in helping people to modify their health behaviors and live longer, healthier lives.

So what is the answer, and what can you do? You might consider offering a CPR and First Aid class in your congregation through the American Red Cross. And you might want to consider purchasing an Automated External Defibrillator (AED) for your congregation and train people to use it.

You could offer a class on heart health to jump start the conversation. The American Heart Association has great materials, such as articles on healthy foods under $1, and DVDs such as "Just a Little Heart Attack," starring Emmy-nominated actress Elizabeth Banks. Health education doesn't have to be boring or expensive.

Make sure everyone knows their numbers—blood pressure, body mass index (BMI), and cholesterol levels. These are important for everyone, but critical for most post-menopausal women, whose bodies will push up their lipids unless they exercise an hour a day. Hosting a health fair would make good sense to help people get screened and to learn about resources for healthy living. On an ongoing basis, help regarding healthy nutrition, exercise, and controlling chronic conditions, such as hypertension and diabetes, will be key.

Foot Care Clinic

QUESTION

I am worried about the feet of some of the parishioners in our congregation and community, particularly older adults with diabetes. I'm thinking of offering a foot clinic in our church. Do you have any suggestions?

With more than 1 out of every 4 adults over 65 living with diabetes (National Diabetes Fact Sheet, 2011) and with other health conditions such as Parkinson's disease or Alzheimer disease also making it difficult for older adults to take care of their feet, this is a valuable service. You are right, however, in that you will want to do this in a way that protects the health of the older adults whose feet may need special care due to vulnerabilities brought about by their health conditions. Sandy Madsen, RN, BSN, education coordinator at Northwest Parish Nurse Ministry, reminds folks that they "do have to be careful with foot care especially when dealing with diabetics and folks with peripheral vascular disease, venous vs. arterial ulcers and the like. Treating feet is quite a specialty, and referral to the correct resource for problems needs to be in the nurse's scope of knowledge. I think it is an excellent idea for the nurse to consider some specialized training."

The Wound, Ostomy and Continence Nursing Certification Board lists programs that include certified foot care education. You may want to consider having someone in your congregation who would be heading this up take one of these classes.

Nancy Moore, RN, parish nurse at Tucker Swamp Baptist Church in Zuni, Virginia, was featured in an issue of *Parish Nurse Perspectives* for her "Sole Care" program. This program was held once a month at the church, with the community invited. Nancy publicized this outreach program in the local newspapers and on the local radio stations in their free broadcast times.

Clients soaked their feet in warm soapy water for fifteen to twenty minutes. This was a time when the "server," or as she called them, "clipper," came to know any clients who were new.

At times, Nancy played soft relaxing background music. Participants also seemed to enjoy gospel music videos. A few regularly came early so they could be with the workers for prayer before they began the ministry session for the day.

Through this ministry, Nancy made referrals to a podiatrist for continued foot care. "What a great feeling to assist people in learning how to care for their feet and to be a part of giving care to a part of the person that is so often not thought about," Nancy said. "Other areas of need have also been discovered and our other ministry teams have come to the rescue! The word of this ministry spread and it is really exciting. The volunteers love it!" The volunteers also provided refreshments during the morning.

Sharon Christensen, RN, MSN, has a similar program for homeless visitors to her downtown Portland parish, St. Andre Bessette Catholic Church. She writes, "I started a foot care ministry after retiring from home health and hospice management in 2004. It has developed into a vibrant ministry with three RNs and volunteers. We have student nurses who help with the program and come back to volunteer. Volunteers wash feet and we have massage tubs after the wash. After that one of the RNs assesses and treats any problems, including consideration of medical problems and looking at the lower extremities. We all believe the treatment that is offered not only is of great assistance and comfort for the homeless but also gives us a chance to spend quality time with these folks and give them advice on other medical conditions and whether or not to seek help from a medical doctor or nurse practitioner. This ministry takes place in the parish, which is situated in downtown Portland, Oregon. None of the RNs have wound, ostomy and continence nursing (WOCN) certification. We have an occasional RN who has a foot care certification."

Blessings to all those who provide care for the whole body, mind, and spirit, and do so in a community-building context! Thanks so much for your interest in offering this program in your setting, as well.

Cancer Programs

QUESTION

Can you recommend any congregational programs that help people living with cancer? I was treated for cancer a while ago, and people with cancer often come to me looking for support.

You have identified one of the key areas of providing support for a person going through such a scary diagnosis as cancer—meeting and talking with someone who has gone through a similar experience and who is willing to talk about it. This is the approach used to help women who have been diagnosed with breast cancer. Often other breast cancer survivors contact them to talk about issues related to their cancer and how their lives are affected.

The church can be a good place to talk about one's worries and situation, because people who receive a diagnosis already know others at church and have a certain level of trust built up. The church can also put into place prayer chains and many helping hands to support a cancer patient with meals, housecleaning, transportation to chemotherapy, and so on. The online network Caring Bridge is another good way to keep people posted about what is happening with someone undergoing treatment in a way that lets the patient or family manage what information is shared.

If the pastor is also willing to preach about the spiritual issues that go along with cancer and other life-threatening illness, such as fear and trust, meaning and purpose, this can be a great comfort. Visits and cards from the pastor or lay people (alone or as a team, depending on the situation and need) can be very helpful and supportive. No one who is part of a church should feel all alone!

Depending on the size and constituents of your congregation, you may find it of value to develop a cancer support group within your congregation or refer folks to support groups elsewhere. Many hospitals have cancer support groups, and there are camps for kids with cancer. One well-known and well-respected family of support groups is Gilda's Clubs (named for the comedian Gilda Radner, who died of ovarian cancer at a relatively young age). They have clubs all around the country and you can find one in your area by searching online for "Gilda's Club." These clubs provide free support to people living with cancer and to their families and friends. You can refer folks to groups like this, or develop your own with elements that are helpful, such as presentations by health providers, social time, and emotional support.

According to the American Cancer Society, about 1.6 million new cancer cases were diagnosed in 2012, not including noninvasive cancer (of any site except urinary bladder) and basal and squamous cell skin cancers. Currently, about 18 million people living in the US have had, or currently have, cancer. This is about 6 percent of the population. Given that churches generally have more older members, the percentage of people you are working with who have cancer may be higher than the national average.

Another part of cancer support is cancer prevention. The American Cancer Society reminds us that all cancers caused by tobacco use and heavy alcohol consumption could be prevented (about 10 percent of all cancer diagnosed). About half of all cancer deaths are from forms of cancer that can be far more easily treated when detected early through screening (colon, rectum, cervix and breast). Also, the Cancer Society states that about one-third of the cancer deaths each year are related to obesity, physical inactivity, and poor nutrition. And protecting the skin from sun and tanning damage could prevent many of the more than two million skin cancers diagnosed annually. Your success as a health educator (for example, with articles on sunscreen or samples available at coffee hour) could prevent many of the cancers of the future.

Whether a cancer might have been prevented or not, all a person with cancer needs is your support. The church must be a place where that support is provided from all quarters.

Stress Education

QUESTION

Could you provide advice on how to write a newsletter article on how stress can interfere with health and wholeness? I'd also like ideas on ways to reduce stress in our lives.

Stress certainly can interfere with health and wholeness in our lives, although as we know, some forms of stress (like riding an exciting ride at Disneyland or going on a travel adventure abroad), are good for most of us during most of our lives.

Stress is inherent in many aspects of our daily lives today. People are living longer, so there is a lot more caregiving going on at the end of our lives. Millions of people live with the stress of serving as an unpaid caregiver for aging loved ones. Chronic and terminal illness brings stress. Our work lives are filled with competing demands, including the explosion of online communications. Our children are programmed to the max, because we fear that our communities are not safe places for them to roam on their own (and in many cases they are not safe). The reasons for stress are as varied as the people who live with those stressors.

In your article, you will of course want to discuss the wide range of negative health effects of stress, which include physical effects such as headaches, muscle tension or pains, stomach aches, chest pains, sleep problems, fatigue, and changes in libido. Emotional effects can include anxiety, restlessness, lack of motivation or focus, irritability or anger, and sadness or depression, and behavior effects can include over- or under-eating, substance abuse and social withdrawal. The Mayo Clinic's website has helpful information about the effects of stress.

Then you will want to explore options for dealing with stress. These include exercise, eating more healthy foods, reducing intake of caffeine, nicotine, alcohol and other mood-altering substances, socializing with friends, taking a vacation or break (even two-minute breaks during the day help), and asking for help, which may come from many places depending on the source of the stress. For example, a person with small children may need your help in finding a mothers' day out program. A person who has just lost a job may need a networking mentoring circle. Someone whose child has a mental illness may need counseling themselves. An individual who has just been diagnosed with a serious illness may need the listening ear of friends or someone to be with them at medical appointments.

Other options for dealing with stress are myriad: going for a walk, prayer or meditation, a bike ride, talking with a mental health professional, a massage, doing Tai Chi, aromatherapy, going for a ten-minute run, taking a break for a cup of herbal tea, joining a choir, playing on a softball team, working on an art project, walking the dog, gardening, swimming, deep breathing, talking with a friend, going to a concert, reading a novel to take your mind off your own problems (since every novel has a problem!), signing up for a Zumba class, acupuncture, going dancing.

Notice how many of these options involve movement. Notice how few involve watching TV or looking at our computers or cell phones. Notice how many involve getting out and being with others. Notice how many involve stopping and doing something else. Some simply involve stopping, like prayer. Blessings to you as you help your congregation respond to stress in healthy ways!

Mental Health

QUESTION
Do you have suggestions for how to approach the topic of mental illness within faith communities?

This is a critical issue. Having the faith community address it takes away much of the stigma and can provide needed support for those living with mental illness and their loved ones. It is necessary to speak out about mental illness, help provide information about resources in the community, and be welcoming to people who are dealing with mental health concerns and their families. As stated by the National Alliance on Mental Illness (NAMI),

> Religious communities are in a unique position to combat stigma and provide a message of acceptance and hope. Proclaiming the values of social justice, respect for all persons, and non-discrimination, faith communities reach out to individuals and families affected by mental illness in many helpful ways. The faith community is the place for content, support and discussion centered around value of spirituality in the recovery process.

You might want to begin online by visiting the website of the National Alliance on Mental Illness, which has a page specifically for faith communities. You will find a listserve to connect with others (NAMI FaithNet), their newsletter, discussion groups, and other links and resources.

Your congregation might consider sponsoring an educational program on a topic of interest, such as eating disorders, suicide prevention, depression, anxiety, bipolar disorder, or any number of other topics related to mental health. Visit the website of the American Association of Pastoral Counselors to locate providers who might be speakers. Or talk to other clergy and faith community nurses in your area for recommendations. Many mental health professionals will be willing to speak with a group in your congregation pro bono or for a small fee. Also, see the winter 2012 issue of *Church Health Reader* which focused on ways churches can address mental illness within their walls and their communities.

Advance Directives

QUESTION

Recently, several of our elderly church members died in the hospital, when I suspect they would rather have died at home. How can I educate the congregation further about advance directives?

Your suspicions may have some real merit. In a study published in the *Annals of Internal Medicine*, researchers found that those patients who had an advance health care directive were more likely to die at home than were those patients who did not have an advance health care directive. ("Brief Communication: The Relationship between Having a Living Will and Dying in Place." Howard B. Degenholtz, PhD; YongJoo Rhee, MPH, PhD; and Robert M. Arnold, MD, *Ann Intern Med*. 20 July 2004;141(2):113-117).

And most people want to die at home—about 70 percent, according to some studies. Yet about 70 percent of deaths in this country now occur in hospitals or other institutions. About 30 percent of people now die in hospitals and about 40 percent in nursing homes.

Most of the rest of us die at home. So how do you improve your chances of having a good death, with only the interventions that you choose? First, you have to be able *to choose*. And in order to choose, you need to tell people while you are still *able to* choose, and the best way to do that involves *writing it down*, along with choosing a health care proxy who can speak for you when you can't.

April 16 is National Healthcare Decisions Day, and I urge you to visit the website of the national initiative by this name (NHDD.org). They have a phenomenal number of materials you can download and use, from fact sheets to videos, to newsletter articles and more.

NHDD.org also has links to organizations where you can get copies of templates for advance directives that are helpful for your state. One outstanding example is Five Wishes, which is comprehensive and also has a guide for training others how to use the Five Wishes document. Other organizations linked from the NHDD include a wide variety of other organizations that provide free state-specific advance directives, from Caring Connections to the MedicAlert Foundation.

It is important to note, however, that Emergency Medical Technicians (EMTs) cannot honor living wills or medical powers of attorney or health care proxy. If 911 is called, EMTs must stabilize and transport a person to a hospital, whether it be from an accident scene or from a private home or other facility. Only a Physician-Ordered Life Sustaining Treatment (POLST) form, which is completed by a physician in consultation with a patient and signed by both, can be followed by EMTs, as the form constitutes "doctor's orders." Also note that not all states have POLST protocols in place. The POLST form is of no use if an EMT can't find it. Put this brightly colored form on the fridge, or the back of the front door, and keep another copy in your wallet or purse. POLST forms, when completed by a physician and signed by the patient, are entered into a database that can be checked by the EMT for verification of the orders on the form.

The same is true for an advance health care directive. It needs to be where people know where it is, so make several copies. Give one to your doctor, one to each of your responsible loved ones, and one to your health care proxy if you have one.

Finally, it makes good sense to schedule a really knowledgeable speaker to come to your church to talk about this, whether it be a hospital chaplain, an elder-law attorney, or someone who makes this the focus of their professional work. This would be a great activity for National Healthcare Decisions Day.

We *all* want to keep the right to choose as long as we possibly can—if possible until death do us part!

CHAPTER 6

Community Engagement

Health Disparities

QUESTION

Our community is very racially divided. I'm not sure what to do about it, but I see the disparity in health as a place to start. Is there anything I should read or consider before doing anything?

Health disparity, as you know, means "difference" related to health, and can be interpreted in several ways. According to the National Institutes of Health (NIH), these differences "can affect how frequently a disease affects a group, how many people get sick, or how often the disease causes death. Many different populations are affected by disparities. These include racial and ethnic minorities; residents of rural areas; women; children; the elderly; and persons with disabilities."

You are correct to note that racial disparities can negatively affect a community, particularly around incidence of certain types of health conditions. For example, according to the National Center for Health Statistics (NCHS), African-Americans have the highest rate of high blood pressure of all racial and ethnic groups, and tend to develop it at younger ages than others.

The target of Healthy People 2010, a program of the US Department of Health and Human Services, was to eliminate disparities by now. Yet, rather than lowering the bar, Healthy People 2020 has raised it by reminding us that one's health status can be impacted by a number of factors. There are disparities in many areas affecting health, including access to a high-quality education; nutritious food; decent and safe housing; affordable and reliable public transportation; culturally sensitive health care providers; access to affordable health insurance; as well as community-wide clean water and non-polluted air.

The NIH has a comprehensive online collection of articles and data about racial and other health disparities online. There you will learn that differences in the health of racial or ethnic groups can result from genetics, environmental factors, access to care, as well as cultural factors. You will also find links to data from the Centers for Disease Control and Prevention (CDC), as well as other governmental and health organizations, sorted by group.

For example, if you click on "Hispanic or Latino Populations," you will link to the Office of Minority Health and Health Disparities (OMHD). There you will find an overview of demographics, leading causes of death, high prevalence health issues, health disparities, and health statistics. They have a host of brochures, slides, and other governmental resources, along with links to non-governmental resources and funders. Of course you will also find a number of resources available in Spanish there, but not as many as you would like, so you will want to click on the "non-governmental resources" and scroll through them to find groups like the National Alliance for Hispanic Health, which has a huge number of resources available in Spanish.

Finally, you will want to call or visit the education department at your local hospital or your public health department. Much of the data related to racial disparities in your community will be available there.

Health Care Missions

QUESTION

I would like to organize our health ministry to offer a health care mission trip outside the country, but I don't know how to start.

You are in good company! A study of faith community nurse vocations found that a common theme among those who were involved in health ministry was an interest in serving for a shorter or longer time in an international setting of need.

The best way to set up a health care mission trip is to partner with a group that has already had experience facilitating this type of work. When working through your church, the easiest place to start is through your denomination. For example, the General Board of Global Ministries of the United Methodist Church has health care volunteer opportunities listed online. They have been doing this for many years and can connect you with programs in other countries that need help. There are many others, such as the Catholic Medical Mission Board and the United Church of Christ/Disciples of Christ partnership.

Denominations may also have more informal ways to partner with sister institutions in other countries. Deborah Goldfeder is a registered nurse (and faith community nurse) who also has a Master of Divinity degree. She and Rev. Susan Naylor (another RN who is an ordained deacon), are both Episcopalians who have had a passion to serve through their denomination in war-torn Sudan, a country that is grossly underserved in health care. They have made several trips to learn, to teach, and to serve through their denomination, working through their local diocese.

Of course, there are other groups with whom you can connect, such as Doctors Without Borders, and organization that includes nurses and other health professionals. The Global Health Council may also be able to connect you with other organizations seeking volunteers.

One particularly good organization that can help groups with varying skills connect as needed in other countries is International Partners in Mission. This organization, based in Ohio, has offices in Europe, Latin America, Asia, and Africa. Founded by returning Lutheran missionaries who felt that mission should be a partnering rather than patronizing, this 35-year old organization can also accommodate those who are not health professionals in their mission efforts.

Another way to serve through foreign mission is to raise funds for an international cause that is badly needed. For example, Dr. Lewis Wall is a practicing Christian and an OG-GYN who specializes in surgery on older women at Washington University School of Medicine and Barnes Hospital in St. Louis, but who also serves in West Africa. He and his wife Helen have raised funds to build a hospital in Niger to help women of all ages who have had a birth trauma injury (fistula). Their hospital is now up and running, and they have a list online of ways to help provide these needed surgeries to women who are needlessly suffering.

Don't forget that there are plenty of opportunities to serve the underserved in this country, as well. Volunteers in Medicine is a great place to get started if you want to explore this option more.

Starting a Dental Clinic

QUESTION

Could you give me some suggestions about starting a dental clinic for people with very little if any money and no insurance?

You have identified a grave need in our communities, as most people in health care, ministry, and social services today know. More than 100 million people in the United States have no dental insurance. And regular dental care is important to overall health. Many of us have experienced firsthand how agonizing a dental emergency can be, and without regular dental care, these can happen far too often. Infections in teeth and gums can spread to the bloodstream and cause severe infection elsewhere. These infections have sometimes tragically caused the death of an adult or child.

There are several models in congregations and communities for offering services, and all of them will take quite a bit of time and effort to make happen. Here are some ways that congregations and communities have made dental care available to people in their neighborhoods:

- Arrange transportation to subsidized or free dental care. Sometimes there are dentists affiliated with federally qualified health centers, dental schools, or other organizations who will see patients for low or no fees, but people can't get there. One solution would be to arrange for transportation from the church to the clinic.

- Arrange for subsidized or free dental care to drive to the church. The "Tooth Taxi" service was created through a partnership with the Oregon Education Association's Choice Trust, ODS Health (a health insurance company) and the Dental Foundation of Oregon. The Tooth Taxi spends up to a week at a time in school districts, and it might be possible for congregations to coordinate with their local schools. Call your school nurses to check if there is a similar program in your area.

- Work with a group such as America's Dentist Care Foundation to set up a dental fair in your community.

- "Just Get It Done Dental Care." When Susan Naylor was the faith community nurse at Centenary United Methodist Church in downtown St. Louis, she noted the need for dental care among many of the refugees who had recently resettled in the area. Through a lot of phone calls, prayer, begging (and did I say praying?), she managed to locate a used dental chair and other needed equipment, and then started calling for donated dental services to serve those in need.

- Affiliate with a free health clinic in another congregation. Some congregations, such as the Alliance Church in Salem, Oregon, have started free health clinics, and dental care is part of the service provided. Call the other churches in your area to see who might already be doing something that you might tap into.

- Build a first-class dental clinic. The Herbert Hoover Boys and Girls Club in St. Louis decided to build a dental clinic for the kids they served in their facility. Their initiative involved a lot of fundraising and grant writing, but they were able to build a small (two-chair) state-of-the-art dental clinic that served the children who belonged to the Boys and Girls Club.

While this is one of the hardest programs to provide through congregations because of the special equipment and skills needed, it is also one of the most needed, so please do prayerfully proceed!

Blood Drives

QUESTION

We are having a hard time recruiting folks for our congregation's twice-yearly blood drive. Do you have any suggestions on how we might excite people to be involved in this important health service?

Blood drives are a great way to help others who need any of the various blood products that are obtained this way, and each donation may help up to three people. But did you know that blood donors may be improving their own health as well? You might try making an announcement like this (or putting something like this in your congregation's newsletter or e-mail blast):

> I am here to offer you an opportunity to reduce your risk of heart disease and save a life at the same time. According to research published in the American Journal of Epidemiology, blood donors are 88 percent less likely to suffer a heart attack and 33 percent less likely to suffer any type of cardiovascular event. Why is that?
>
> One theory is blood donors are generally more healthy people. They must be free of a number of health conditions to be considered as a donor, so this may be a self-selected healthier group. Another theory is that donating a pint of blood removes a small amount of iron from your circulatory system, which may reduce your risk for hardening of the arteries (atherosclerosis).
>
> In addition, you can lose a pound in just a few minutes! What's not to love about this way to help save a life (maybe even your own)?

Just a quick note: the need for blood donation rises at certain times of the year, such as summers when schools and colleges who hold blood drives are out of session. And the whole process from your welcoming sign-in to a guilt-free cookie takes only about an hour (and the actual blood draw takes only about 10 minutes).

Try to recruit people to recruit their friends directly. People are more likely to do something if someone asks them directly than if they just read a note about it. Your whole health committee may need to make some personal calls. And you should be equipped to answer a lot of questions. Luckily, the American Red Cross makes the answers to most of those questions readily available on their website. First-time donors may wonder what tests are done during screening, what questions they are asked, whether the process is painful, or how often they can donate blood.

You might also try a theme for your blood drive. Some themes folks have used in the past include holiday themes, seasonal themes, sports themes (think baseball!), nautical, and Mardi Gras, among others. The American Red Cross also has a list of great ideas for blood drive event themes online.

And thanks for your efforts on behalf of all those in the communities you serve!

Cooling Center

QUESTION

We'd like to open a cooling center for our older adults or people with disabilities that might be suffering from the heat in their homes. Do you have any suggestions for how our health ministry team might do that?

Good for you for taking a team approach to this important effort through your health ministry team! And if you don't have a health ministry team, do assemble a committee to explore this idea as soon as possible, because it would be impossible to do this alone. (Well, with God all things are possible, but none of us is God!)

Here are some questions for you to consider with your committee:

Would you be open only for church members or for anyone from the community? Your question indicates that you would like to open this to the full community, but be sure to get buy-in from the leadership and the congregation before you proceed, because this is a bigger task than it appears. On average, serving 20 people or so for a week will take more than 70 volunteers, serving two meals a day.

Who will decide when the temperature is hot enough that it warrants the center to be opened? In Oregon, centers are opened when the temperature hits 90 degrees in the summer, but that certainly wouldn't be hot enough for Missouri to open its cooling shelters.

What hours are you able to be open for guests? You certainly would need to offer different services for daytime and nighttime shelter.

What facilities do you have available to make your guests comfortable during the day? How many restrooms do you have available? Who will monitor them for cleanliness for your guests?

What facilities do you have available to make your guests comfortable overnight? Do you have showers available? A place to do laundry if folks are stuck there for a few days? Do you have cots? Bedding? Towels? You probably will want to have at least two overnight hosts from the church—a man and a woman—for each night.

What about food? Are you able to offer snacks or meals or can you arrange for a food cart or carts to sell meals in your parking lot? If meals or snacks are being offered through the congregation, who will be in charge of each meal? Do you have a caterer in your church who could arrange for meals at short notice?

What about security? How can you both be welcoming and keep the sanctuary a safe space for all?

How will you communicate that your congregation is available to serve the community in this way? You might want to be in conversation with your local health department, Red Cross, and area agencies on aging, for example, to let them know about your intention to help.

Would you be willing to extend your shelter for other purposes? For example, could your church basement be used as a shelter from severe storms? What about other emergencies? Here is where being in good communication with your public health officials would be a real asset.

How many church members does it take to change a lightbulb? Only one, but it needs to be the person who knows where the light bulbs are—and the ladder. Be sure to recognize and honor your building steward for the extra effort this takes on that person too!

Veteran Support

QUESTION

How can our health ministry committee provide support for veterans returning from war zones and for their families?

Good for your church in providing support to veterans. Your health committee can help in a number of ways.

Make sure to provide all the services with privacy and dignity. This may mean that you might meet with the veteran's spouse, if requested, or you might travel to meet with the family at their home rather than at the church. Ask what would be helpful to them, and don't presume. Listen.

Here is a sampling of areas of potential need in reintegrating into civilian life after returning from deployment:

- Help with understanding health care benefits and advocating for needed services. For example, returning vets may have access to dental care and to several years of free health care. A health committee member can be an advocate to help navigate the VA system to access needed services. Sometimes simply being available to talk can encourage the veteran to "hang in there" to persevere in getting to the right services.
- Can the church provide trained and screened babysitters who would be willing to care for children for a time in the evening to give the parents a break?
- Is there someone who can help a veteran navigate the admissions process at a local college?
- Who might have affordable housing available for a returning military family?
- Who might have work available for a veteran or a member of the veteran's family?
- Is someone a qualified auto mechanic who could help with car repairs or help the family to find a reliable car?
- Would someone with a truck farm be willing to give a share of the crop each week to help the family?
- Is there a need for a mother's group at the church to help families make friends after a move?
- Is there a need for a safe space for recreation and fellowship, like a Saturday morning pick-up basketball game, or a softball league team?
- Can the health committee put together a mini-directory for veterans of who might be willing to do what to help?

This list is just a sampling of what might be needed or helpful to returning veterans and their families. Being welcoming and prepared by talking about this in advance with your congregation will go a long way to making the church a place that can help military families re-enter the community in a healing and helpful way.

Housing

QUESTION

Our health committee and mission outreach committee would like to find a way to work together on a project. Can you suggest something that might fit the intent of each of these committees?

Access to safe and affordable housing might be an area where the mission of both of your committees could converge, combining hands-on service opportunities and advocacy with the documented health benefits of permanent housing.

For example, Habitat for Humanity has been building homes to help low-income families for many years. Much of its work has been in partnership with faith communities, but it has lost traction with faith communities lately. It's time to take another look at this important mission through the lens of health ministry.

Why health ministry? The health benefits of home ownership are well documented. According to the archive at Human Impact Partners, articles providing evidence-based support for safe, affordable housing make these claims:

- Improved access to neighborhoods with health-promoting assets, such as grocery stores, places to exercise, good schools
- Lower child unintentional injury rates
- Higher self-esteem and more positive mental health
- Children are more likely to graduate from high school, a strong indicator for later improved health as compared to those who do not complete high school.
- Traditionally, homes have appreciated in value, adding to the financial stability of the family. Financial health is positively co-related to physical health due to increased access to healthy lifestyles and quality medical care.

So how can you get involved?

- Call your local chapter of Habitat for Humanity and jump in on the building of a house, or raise money to help support the building of a house.
- Check with local women's shelters about the need for transitional housing for women after they leave the shelters. Lydia's House in St. Louis was started in 1994 by two clergywomen and two laywomen to provide housing up to two years as women seek employment to build up a nest egg for home ownership. Today, what started with one house serves up to 35 families at a time.
- Work with an organization such as the Salem Interfaith Hospitality Network, which provides food and shelter for families in congregations, rotating a week at a time. The network also provides support to these families in the process of qualifying for and obtaining permanent housing. Last year this organization helped 52 families move into permanent housing—that's one every week! Each congregation has sign-ups for the various tasks that need to be done each day. Currently, 900 people volunteer to help with this program, such as bringing a side dish for a dinner, or serving as a host for an evening.
- You might find ways to help people who are in trouble with their mortgages or being discriminated against in seeking housing. There is a huge racial disparity in home ownership, with more than 75 percent of whites owning homes, and fewer than 50 percent of African Americans and Latinos owning homes.

While housing isn't a health issue in the same way as taking someone's blood pressure, it certainly does have an impact on the well-being of an entire family. Also, there are plenty of ways to get involved, from hands-on building to helping in the gap.

Health Ministry Advice for Everyone

Senior Housing

QUESTION

Our church is thinking about building some church-related housing for seniors. Is this idea fesible? Where should we look for information?

The seniors in your community are not alone in their need. According to the National Council on Aging, only one federal program provides housing for low-income seniors (Section 202), and the average resident in that program is 79 years old with an income below $10,000. For every unit that becomes available, ten seniors are on the waiting list.

Developing senior housing, however, is something that is possible in any area. There are a wide variety of options for moving forward, and most include community partnerships. One on the small end is the example of Josephburg United Church of Canada, which has fewer than 100 members. They partnered with the tiny community in which they were located (Josephburg, Alberta, population 234), to build a four-unit apartment building for local seniors. At the other end of the spectrum, Beatitudes United Church of Christ in Phoenix, Arizona built a continuing care retirement community (CCRC) known as Beatitudes Campus of Care. This facility has a range of housing options for several hundred people, including some private subsidies, although no government subsidies (they are not part of Section 202 funding). They serve the "broad middle class," and this demographic includes the majority of seniors.

Beatitudes's story is compelling. The pastor of their young congregation, Rev. Bill Nelson, was appalled by the housing options available for seniors, and the congregation gave money to build Beatitudes Campus of Care before they built their sanctuary. It took many folks working together to address zoning issues and other challenges, but the first residents moved in within three years of the original decision to build. Beatitudes now has skilled nursing, assisted living, and several hundred independent living apartments.

Still other congregations have worked with faith-based organizations such as the Retirement Housing Foundation (RHF) to focus on housing for those who have very modest incomes. RHF is one of the nation's largest non-profit providers of low-income housing for older adults and persons with disabilities. It was founded more than 50 years ago (1961) by two clergy and a layman, with $7,000 between them raised for this purpose. They now provide many thousands of housing units in more than half of all US states.

So start doing market research. What is available in your community, what are the occupancy rates, how long are waiting lists, and what type of fees do they charge? Talk to folks in your congregation and community about whether they would get involved. If you confirm the need and uncover interest in participating, then form a committee, including clergy and laity who have experience working with housing, government or social services.

Healthy Food Pantry

QUESTION

Our food pantry is open a few hours every weekday. Do you have some suggestions on items members could contribute that would be healthier, but not so expensive that the suggestions deter giving?

In these tough economic times, the kindness and generosity of those who contribute to feed the hungry is greatly appreciated, and it's wonderful that your food pantry is open every day. I'm sure it makes a real difference in the lives of many. How good it is that you are thinking about ways to encourage others to share, and to do so in ways that stretch a food budget dollar.

Here are some suggestions for healthy foods that can be donated to food pantries.

- Brown rice is a healthy alternative to canned starches, such as ravioli in tomato sauce. It contains far less sodium, and costs far less per serving.

- Consider substituting whole wheat versions of pasta whenever possible.

- While green beans are cheap, other kinds of beans, such as kidney or garbanzo beans, are far more versatile. They can be used in soups or salads, or baked with a little brown sugar, ketchup, mustard, and vinegar for a tasty dish with brown rice. Rinsing these canned beans in a colander will remove as much as 40 percent of the sodium. Of course, dried beans take a little longer to prepare, but they have no sodium at all.

- Did you know that milk can be frozen? If you are able to get a good buy on milk, and have room to freeze it in your food pantry, this is a good way to provide some protein.

- Tuna packed in water is a good option for protein, and sometimes canned salmon is a good price, too.

- If purchasing soups, look for low-sodium varieties. If purchasing canned fruit or juices, avoid those with added sugar.

- Oatmeal is a good choice for a breakfast cereal donation, along with other low-sugar cereals.

- Peanut butter provides a good amount of protein, and natural peanut butters are the healthiest versions.

- Canned tomatoes are versatile and can be used in pasta sauces, with a variety of meats, and in soups or casseroles. Unfortunately, the canning process for tomatoes still involves BPA (to keep the acid in the tomatoes from eating the can). But for most other vegetables, Environmental Working Group Eden Organic canned goods do not contain BPA.

- Powdered milk fortified with Vitamin D is another healthy choice.

If your church has a way to store and rotate fresh produce, by all means make every effort to do so. You might partner with a neighborhood garden, with a few local gardeners, or with area farmers to provide produce. Or you may buy it in bulk with donations and make individual or family-sized portions available to those who use the food pantry.

Don't forget that items like diapers and toilet paper might also be needed and welcomed.

CHAPTER 7

Church Life and Activities

Movie Nights

QUESTION

Our health team was thinking of sponsoring a movie night at church. Do you have any suggestions for a "Healthy Movie Night?"

What a great idea! There are a number of good movies that might work, particularly for teens and adults. Here are a few suggestions.

- *Supersize Me*—This film was made by independent filmmaker Morgan Spurlock, who tried the experiment of eating every meal at the same fast food chain every day for a month, choosing the healthiest options as often as possible. You'll want to watch to the end to see how he fared.
- *Forks Over Knives*—Lee Fulkerson wrote and directed this film, which is available on DVD. It explores the idea that most of the degenerative diseases that people develop can be controlled or reversed by rejecting our focus on animal-based and processed foods.
- *Food, Inc.*—Filmmaker Robert Kenner explores the corporatization of our food, much of which is controlled (bought, processed, packaged, and distributed) by just a few companies. It provides good food for thought, and a strong argument for growing as much of your own food as you can or supporting your local farmer's market and independent food producers directly.
- *May I Be Frank*—Frank Ferrante, an overweight middle-aged recovering addict, stumbles into the vegan Café Gratitude, where he begins a life-changing journey of learning to care for himself.
- *Babette's Feast*—Unlike some of the movies above, this G-rated movie does not have any bias against eating meat. Its message is more about living as whole people—body, mind, and spirit, in community, and in harmony with creation.

Here are some tips for making your movie night fun.

1. Watch the movie you are going to show yourself so that you are familiar with the plot and the message. Plan discussion questions if you would like to include a discussion as part of the evening or as a follow-up gathering.
2. Make posters to advertise your movie night, and blow them up like movie theater posters. Advertise in all the usual places (bulletin, newsletter, etc.) with a brief synopsis of the movie.
3. Healthy movie snacks might include: popcorn popped in canola oil, fresh fruit cut in bite-sized pieces or dried fruit, low-fat string cheese, fresh raw veggies. Make a yummy dip for fruit with pureed strawberries blended into plain yogurt with a little vanilla and honey. For more ideas, look at page 68.
4. Make an evening of it with dinner and a movie. Plan a healthy meal and get the health team involved in choosing the menu and bringing recipes to share. Clean up the meal before you start the movie, so that everyone can enjoy the fun.
5. Hire qualified childcare workers to watch the younger kids and let them enjoy a movie such as "Babe" or "Charlotte's Web" along with the healthy dinner or snacks.
6. Remember that "sitting is the new smoking," so build a little dancing into the evening with some line-dancing or an "instant recess" as an intermission, or before or after the movie.

If you want to have a movie series, assign different folks on the committee to preview each movie and introduce it for that evening. Solicit ideas along the way for other movies that might fit the theme. Maybe you have a resident expert on film or food in your congregation or community who would like to say a few words before the film (emphasis on *few*).

Be aware that there will be different points of view about the movie, and that's okay. That's what movies are for—to entertain and to make us consider what we think.

Health Ministry Advice for Everyone

Fundraisers

QUESTION

The Christmas bazaar committee is asking new groups to get involved. We want to stay true to our mission as a health team, yet help them raise funds. Do you have any ideas?

Here is a way that you might get someone new involved in providing items for the bazaar, along with providing health benefits to the congregation, community, and the earth. Why not invite an experienced beekeeper to speak to an adult education class about beekeeping in your area? Entice someone to raise bees and bring honey to sell at the bazaar. You can find a speaker through the magazine *Bee Culture* or contact your local state university's extension department for a recommendation. If you start early in the year, you will be able to collect honey in time to sell when the bazaar comes along.

You may not want to have a beehive at the church where children can get into it, or where it alarms someone who might be allergic to bee stings. More likely you will interest a couple of people to do this at home as a hobby and donate some of their honey to the Christmas bazaar.

Before you completely dismiss the idea of hives at the church, however, you should know that many urban areas are perfect settings for hives on rooftops. Planning and maintenance make this possible in almost any urban setting. An experienced beekeeper should be able to help. For example, bees need plenty of fresh water nearby, or they will go looking for it. Also, colonies divide (swarm) after their first winter, so you will need to keep making room in the hive and set up swarm traps in the trees nearest the hives. Again, an experienced beekeeper can help. Finally, new beekeepers need to learn how to safely process their honey.

What are the benefits? First, there is the financial benefit to the bazaar, which relates to the original question. What does a pound of honey cost? You can probably ask between $5.00 to $8.00 a pound for honey, and selling it in nice one-pound honey bears with a holiday ribbon would be a festive bazaar treat.

There are also health benefits to honey. It seems to work well as a cough suppressant (but should not be given to children under one year of age), has some antioxidant properties, and can be used as a topical anti-inflammatory for mosquito bites, among other claims.

Then there are the health benefits to the earth of keeping bees. Colony collapse disorder has cause the demise of many colonies, and replenishing the bees of the earth is a great way to help the health of gardens and fields near the hives.

Beekeeping isn't for everyone, and it takes planning ahead. But if someone would like to give it a try, it might be a healthful and helpful way to make a contribution to the Christmas bazaar that would last the whole year long.

Quilting

QUESTION

Our quilting group has been involved in our church's health ministry through making prayer quilts, and would like to expand our outreach. Do you have any ideas for what we might do?

You might want to try what has been done at Coffee Creek, a women's correctional facility in Wilsonville, Oregon. In 2002, Koko Sutton had the idea of a starting a quilting program there and began to recruit volunteers. Ten years later, they now have 20 sewing machines and four weekly classes, each with five volunteer instructors and 20 students.

On average, the program at Coffee Creek generates about 150 quilts per year. Each student designs and makes two quilts to give away to a charity such as hospice or teen shelters. The third quilt each person makes through the program is hers to keep.

The program is a gift to the community. Here is what one daughter of a quilt recipient said: "My mother was a patient at Portland's Legacy Emanuel Hospital. When we knew we were losing Mama, the hospital chaplain brought the beautiful quilt, telling us that it was called a 'passage quilt.' We kept our mother covered with this beautiful quilt as she was dying, and we proudly displayed it at her funeral service."

And the program is a gift to the women who participate, as well. Here is what one of the program participants said about making a quilt: "The quilting program was the first time I felt good about myself since being in prison. When I finished that first quilt, I began feeling better about myself and having some self-confidence. I never finished anything before."

The cost of the program is approximately $100 per participant per year. Funds are donated by congregations, groups such as Thrivent Financial for Lutherans, other quilters' groups, and craft shops. Overflow storage for the program is in donated space at a local church, and the volunteers bring supplies as needed.

Upon release from prison, and after successful reintegration into a home situation, each former inmate may request a release kit, which includes a refurbished service sewing machine, sewing supplies, patterns, and so on. The exchange is made in a public place, neither at the home of the former inmate nor at the home of the volunteer.

For more information, visit the website of the Coffee Creek Quilters. They offer a guide that tells how to go about starting a quilting program in a correctional facility, along with the policies and procedures for training, screening, and safety.

Quilting really can heal lives!

Presenting Prayer Shawls

QUESTION

Do you have any advice for how to present a prayer shawl to a large group? We have 25 prayer shawls to present to our confirmation class and I am puzzled regarding the best way to do this. Any suggestions?

Twenty-five kids in your confirmation class? Wow! Those prayers must be getting answered! All kidding aside, those prayer shawls will be a wonderful symbol to your confirmation class. One faith community nurse told me about how her congregation presented prayer shawls to their graduating seniors. They had been receiving feedback about how much the students, most of whom now were attending university, appreciated the gift from their congregation—a warm and tender reminder of home.

You have a variety of options. One is to arrange for each of the prayer shawls to be presented by the person who made it, and have the person say a short prayer of blessing, as he or she places the prayer shawl on the confirmand. Presenters may say something like, "May the love of God surround you and bless you all of your days." Or you might have the giver recite a Bible verse as they place the prayer shawl on the young person. It would be very nice if you had 25 different people make and present the prayer shawls so that each confirmand could be connected to the person who made the shawl for him or her. If that is not possible, or if you would rather not say who made each one, you could have the prayer shawl presented by the minister or a parent.

Another option is to present a prayer shawl to each, and then say a prayer for all of them together, something like this:

God of peace and blessing, we pray that you would surround these young people, your blessed children, with wisdom and courage, love and grace. Help them to feel the presence of this gathered community on this, their confirmation day. Help them to know that we will be with them and support them in all that they do. Help them to choose the right. In the years that lie ahead, strengthen them in faith, guide them in your paths, fill them with the knowledge of your saving love, and help them to find their true purpose in your glorious creation. This we pray in your holy name. Amen.

A note for churches who don't have knitters: prayer quilts are nice, too!

Choir

QUESTION

What about the people in choir? Is there some way to involve them in health ministry? They are already committed one evening a week, and on Sundays before services as well.

The choir members in your church are already involving you in their health ministry, and have been for as long as they have been singing with the choir. "What are you talking about," you ask?

There seems to be good data that supports the positive health effects of singing, from increasing one's lung capacity and oxygen exchange, to releasing endorphins that increase one's well-being. (Whether a particular singer is capable of increasing someone else's well-being is open to question, but we are called to "make a joyful noise," so hopefully the rest of the choir will balance out the off-key bellower.) When you join the choir in singing the hymns, you too can experience this positive effect on your own health. Thanks to the faithful choir for leading the congregation in song!

In addition, there is data that shows that song can connect with folks who have difficulty with communication, such as people with autism or dementia, such as Alzheimer disease. Certainly, music therapists have experienced this on a daily basis, but one need not be a music therapist to provide the benefit of song. After seeing the positive response of people in residential care to song in 2002, Chreanne Montgomery-Smith, in West Berkshire, UK, founded "Singing for the Brain" and started weekly singing sessions for people with Alzheimer disease.

There is also good data that supports the positive health effects of being active in a community. Loneliness is a leading risk factor for illness, so the choir member who is expected to be somewhere one evening every week and then come back again every Sunday, both before and during services, is less likely to experience loneliness than someone who has no regular commitments. And a church choir is generally a place where all are welcomed, if not begged, to join.

Having said that, we all know the expression, "It ain't over 'til the fat lady sings," and it is clear that one can be dreadfully overweight or obese and still be a fine singer, even a major opera star. More and more, however, the outstanding singers of our day are people who take seriously the importance of keeping one's whole body strong and healthy, not just one's throat and lungs.

What to do? Here are seven ideas to get you started.

- Invite a physician or nurse in your congregation to come talk with the choir about healthy practices that can improve their stamina and help them protect their voices.

- Invite a visiting artist or music educator to talk with the choir about their own health practices as a role model.

- Invite choir members to come to Sunday school or other children's activities and lead vocal exercises for fun.

- Invite the "vocal athletes" in your church to present a class to adult education or the women's or men's fellowship in which they demonstrate the physical aspects of singing (along with an invitation to join the choir).

- Consider starting a "Singing for the Brain" type of program in your church for members and friends living with Alzheimer disease.

- Have choir members lead a "sing-along" movie night with a good musical, such as "Sound of Music," as part of a youth "lock-in" or a family night.

- Sponsor a "Talent Night" as a fundraiser for your health ministry program and invite choir members and other musical types to perform.

Unfortunately, as a former church choir director myself, I can tell you from experience that the choir members are probably not going to be the first to sign up for health ministry programs. But if you can appeal to their love of music and performance, you can get them, too, involved in health ministries.

Labyrinths

QUESTION

We are planning to create a labyrinth, but I'd love for it to have another purpose as well than only spiritual reflection. Do you have any ideas?

Most of God's creation has more than one purpose—a river can be beautiful while providing a home for fish, water for our crops, and quenching thirst in our own bodies. A labyrinth can offer various benefits as well. Of course, the spiritual benefits alone from a labyrinth are many, and I won't go into them here. But here are some suggestions for you as you think about multiplying the ministries of your labyrinth together with others in your congregation.

- **Turn your labyrinth into a memorial garden to provide solace to the grieving.** Invite family members to donate bricks or paving stones with the names of their loved ones to place along the path to be remembered by those who walk the labyrinth. Check with local companies who do engraving or search online for "engraved bricks," but remember the additional cost for bricks that must be shipped. These bricks can be sold as a fundraiser for your grief support ministry.

- **Use herbs of the Bible to create the labyrinth.** Obviously, not all herbs mentioned in the Bible will grow outdoors in all climates, but if your labyrinth passes near a church window, some of the more tender herbs can be grown indoors in the cooler climates. Also, the herbs can be dried and sold at the church bazaar, or can be used in cooking meals for the hungry. Here are some of the herbs that you might consider: coriander (Exodus 16:31), cumin (Matthew 23:23), mint (Matthew 23:23), dill (Matthew 23:23), garlic (Numbers 11:5), and mustard (Matthew 13:31). Notice how several of them are very hardy indeed—a wonderful metaphor for God's persistent love! Be sure to label the various plantings and include the Scripture verse in which they are mentioned.

- **Plant healing plants of the Bible in the labyrinth.** For example, the aloe plant (Proverbs 7:17) is useful for treating minor burns. Mint (Matthew 23:23) made into tea calms nausea and helps quiet the bowels. Mustard (Matthew 13:31) has been used for mustard plasters to treat respiratory illnesses for many years. And chamomile (Isaiah 40:6) is made into a restorative tea. Like the herbs above, be sure to label the plantings and include the Scripture verse in which they can be found.

- **Plant vegetables and fruit in the labyrinth.** Consider a labyrinth planting with vegetables and perhaps a fruit tree—perhaps apple—in the middle. In the labyrinth at St. Elizabeth Ann Seaton in Aloha, Oregon, parish nurse Sally Perry and others planted a well-planned garden with a wide variety of vegetables, including lettuce, spinach, chard, collard greens, carrots, radishes, parsnips, peas, chilies, bell peppers, eggplant, cabbage, sweet corn, pole beans, summer and winter squash, pumpkins, onions, and a wide variety of tomatoes. The taller plants were around the outside, moving inwards toward the lettuce and other leafy green plants at the middle.

- **Enlarge your labyrinth and plant trees.** Do a wonderful thing for the earth and plant trees around your labyrinth to remove carbon dioxide from the atmosphere and generate oxygen for those of us creatures that breathe instead of living through photosynthesis. Contact your local nursery for advice on trees that will work in such a setting.

- **Make a play labyrinth with sand and grass.** Children of all ages will love walking in bare feet through the labyrinth. Slowly walking in sand with bare feet is very good for the balance. You might combine some time with this labyrinth for older adults with a Tai Chi class.

Put your imagination (and that of your health committee's) to work, and I'm sure you can come up with several more ideas.

Chronic Illness Support Groups

QUESTION

I keep hearing from people who have dropped out of chronic illness support groups because the people they see there are sicker than they are. Do you have any advice for how I can do this in a way that would be helpful?

This is a very good question. Support groups may be best for people who have real hope for getting better. Or for people who have real hope. I think these are two different things.

The first—real hope for getting better—works with conditions like alcohol abuse and other addictions, where the group support can offer hope for a better life. It also works for health conditions like breast cancer, where tremendous strides have been made towards cure and there is hope for new cures, as well. And a support group can be helpful for emotionally difficult challenges like caregiving, where a group can offer respite and a reconnection to one's life separate from the person needing care.

A support group seems to be less helpful with health conditions where there is an inexorable road to physical decline. Even if everyone has the same illness, to the newcomer it is readily apparent that others who are further along in the disease really are not a peer group to those who are newly diagnosed.

However, having said that, the church itself is a support group for people who have real hope. No matter what our physical condition, we all hope for what we do not see and take on faith that God's love is eternal. We partake, as embodied spiritual beings, in that eternity while only seeing a part of it in the present. Death and dying (the evidence of which is probably one of the most feared aspects of joining a support group), is an inevitable part of life. This becomes abundantly clear in grief support groups.

Many groups of people can benefit from gathering with others who have like needs and concerns, such as those who are mourning the loss of a spouse, those who are parenting special needs children, those who are waiting to adopt children, those who are trying to lose weight, and so on. Support groups are part of a faith community's toolbox to help others. The University of Kansas has a very helpful online resource entitled, "The Community Tool Box." This has a chapter on creating and facilitating peer support groups, which serve more than six million Americans at any given time.

For health ministers, it is important to decide whether you have the expertise to lead a support group, including both expertise in content and expertise in facilitating the group process. In most cases, you would do well to find an outside facilitator for a topic unless it is your area of expertise. For example, the Alzheimer Café, which provides peer groups for people living with Alzheimer disease and their families, expects that a presentation by an expert on some aspect of this illness be a part of each session for the caregivers. If you are leading a support group as a peer leader, you will need to have some understanding of the issue to be an effective participant on the topic. And if you want to lead a time-limited evidence-based program such as Powerful Tools for Caregivers, you will need to go through the training that will prepare you to offer the program.

Of course, before starting any support group you will want to research the demand for a particular type of group in your church and community. Also look into whether there is a local, regional or national organization working on this topic with which you can connect and turn to for advice, resources, and other support. Don't reinvent the wheel.

When you have chosen a focus, decide whether you want the group to be by invitation only or open to the public, and whether it should meet for a few weeks or months, or on an ongoing basis. Will you charge a small fee to cover the costs of materials or snacks? Who will be in charge of communications, room set-up, and so on? Finally, who will be in charge of facilitating the process of sharing to make sure everyone is included and heard?

Do your homework on the front end, but don't be afraid to change things as you go along. And don't be afraid to reach out to form a support group. After all, isn't gathering the people together for mutual support a big part of what the church is—and always has been—about?

Healing and Hymns

QUESTION

I know that music is an important component of healing, and that the use of familiar hymns can often reach someone with dementia. Do you have any suggestions on the use of hymnody in health ministry?

This topic was the focus of a Lilly sabbatical project that I received through the Louisville Institute, which resulted in the resource, *Balm in Gilead: Hymns of Healing and Wholeness*. While collecting hymns for this resource, along with the stories of their text authors and composers, I was deeply touched by the pain and courage of generations of faithful people who responded to God's presence through the hope and message of music. Each hymn in that resource includes a summary of those stories.

Deborah Carlton Loftis, the executive director of The Hymn Society in the United States and Canada, put together a healing service which focused on hymns. In working on this service, Deborah asked whether singing these hymns might "provide an opportunity for individuals to face the pain they've been trying to squelch and ignore? Could the singing be a chance for the congregation to express their love and acceptance of someone who is hurting? Just as physical wounds have to be cared for so that they heal properly, our emotional and spiritual wounds must be cared for as well. Might these texts provide a window of opportunity to provide the needed care? How could the hymns we sing encourage us to reach out with God's arms to those around us?"

One program that has built on these deep connections of music to healing and wholeness related to dementia is the "Singing for the Brain" program offered through the Alzheimer's Association in the UK. Familiar music can often calm an agitated individual, and there is some evidence that music builds networks in the brain that can be reactivated and soothed when the music is heard again later in life. And often familiar music can trigger some renewed use of language, if only for a moment.

In any case, don't be shy about using music with your health ministry programs. Ask your choir director, choir members, or a local music therapist for help, or do it yourself. Here are some recommended hymns to get you started. You will see their stories are filled with pain, yet trust in God's redeeming love and care. There are many more. Enjoy seeking them out, and singing them with others.

- *Now Thank We All Our God* (written by a pastor after his wife died in the plague)
- *What a Friend We Have In Jesus* (written by a young man in Canada to his mother back in Ireland)
- *It is Well with My Soul* (written by a man who lost all four daughters in a shipwreck)
- *Pass Me Not, O Gentle Savior* (written by Fanny Crosby about a man in prison)
- *Guide My Feet* (African American spiritual, written at a time of great suffering)

Music is for all, whether we sing, hum, tap our toes, weep, or quietly meditate. The hymnody of the church has much healing balm to share with all.

CHAPTER 8

Congregational Care

Dementia

QUESTION

How can we deal with church members who have dementia? Recently two male members almost came to blows due to the behavior of the one with dementia. How could our health ministry help deal with this?

Dementia can take many different forms, with some people just getting confused but retaining their outwardly sweet demeanors and others having what seem to be rather negative changes to their behaviors and interactions with others. These negative impulses could have been there before, but changes in the brain often decrease one's ability to regulate these types of words and actions. It sounds like this is what has happened in the situation you have described.

Dementia is on the rise as people live longer and the large cohort of baby boomers moves into the senior years. According to the Aging, Demographics and Memory Study of the nationally representative Health and Retirement Study (HRS), approximately 13.9 percent of individuals living in their homes over the age of 71 were found to have some level of dementia (as opposed to normal cognition or cognitive impairment without dementia). That's nearly six million people, and it doesn't even include those who are living in residential facilities who have dementia.

It's important to remember there are many causes of dementia, including Alzheimer disease, strokes, head injuries, long-term alcohol abuse, medication side effects or interactions, and other physical illnesses. Dementia can range from mild to severe.

I've broken this down into three questions.

1. **What can be done for the person with dementia?** Try to ensure that he or she is receiving appropriate medical care for illness, and that the person has the ability to live as good a quality of life as possible with this condition. This question includes looking at health and being sure the individual has access to health care providers who can help. Look at the health behaviors (Is the person eating healthy food and sleeping?). Look also at the home environment (Is the fridge full of decaying food? Is the house clean enough to safely live in? Does the person pay bills on time?). Find out who is helping with daily tasks (What are their family and neighborhood supports?). What can be done to help a person with dementia is a *huge* question, and I know you are up to answering it, with the help of family supports, your congregation, and the health care and social service providers in your community.

2. **What can be done for the person who has encountered someone with dementia?** Obviously, if both people are long-time members of the church, the one who does not have dementia may know what is going on with a fellow parishioner—but may not. You are under an ethical obligation as a faith community nurse (and if you were not a health professional you would still be under an ethical obligation as a Christian) to protect and honor the privacy of the health information of the individual with any health condition. Having said that, you can always debrief the one who was wronged by asking what he or she thinks might have been going on and help the person come to a compassionate conclusion.

3. **What can be done for all the members of the faith community?** Education about mental health issues, including dementia, may be one of the most important things you can do for your congregation and community. Invite a speaker from the Alzheimer's Association or someone doing brain research from a nearby university or teaching hospital to speak about the healthy brain and what can go wrong, including brain injuries, strokes, and forms of dementia. You might also support the cognitive well-being of folks through activities which studies have shown to be good for your brain, such as exercise, eating healthy foods, getting enough sleep, socializing, challenging your mind through life-long learning, and managing your medications.

Hoarding

QUESTION

I am a faith community nurse and have helped move an elderly hoarder to a safe environment. There are several more hoarders in our church. How do we approach this? How can we love them enough to make a difference?

I hadn't thought of hoarding as that much of a health problem. Maybe it's denial, as those who have seen my workspace might say! But when I started to research your question, it became clear that for hoarders, this behavior can evolve into serious health and safety issues. In addition, hoarding can lead to profound social and financial difficulties, such as loss of friendships, divorce, eviction, and homelessness.

The Mayo Clinic defines hoarding as "the excessive collection of items, along with the inability to discard them. Hoarding often creates such cramped living conditions that homes may be filled to capacity, with only narrow pathways winding through stacks of clutter. Some people also collect animals, keeping dozens or hundreds of pets often in unsanitary conditions."

According to the International OCD Foundation, the average age of a person seeking help for hoarding seems to be about 50 and as many as 1 in 20 people may be hoarders to various degrees. So it should be no surprise that you have run across several in your congregation.

How do you assist people to get the help they need? One way, as you have found, is to move an elderly person into an environment that is more controlled, such as an assisted living facility where "stuff" is monitored and managed. But younger people, or elderly people who won't agree to move and who retain their own guardianship, will need to be convinced to seek other help for their problem.

Here are four other ways to help:

- **Invite a speaker**. As with most health issues, education is key. Invite a speaker who is knowledgeable about this disorder to make a presentation at the church. You might try contacting the Anxiety and Depression Association of America for names of speakers in your area, or contact your local mental health providers.

- **Increase awareness**. Create a bulletin board about hoarding. Spring cleaning time would be a good season to do this. You can find a helpful fact sheet about hoarding created by the International OCD Foundation from which you can create bulletin board materials (available in English and Spanish). And you can find more helpful information from the ADAA.

- **Explore counseling**. Encourage the person or people about whom you have a concern to talk with a therapist who is experienced with this type of behavior. A skilled therapist can help the person who is hoarding learn how to get rid of clutter by dealing with the underlying issues, help find a support group, and help develop a plan to prevent future hoarding. There are both outpatient and in-patient treatment options available, and depending on the provider, the cost may be covered by private insurance, Medicare, or Medicaid. The Mayo Clinic, for example, accepts all these forms of payment. Other clinics only accept self-pay, so be sure you check this out. The International OCD Foundation offers a list on their website of clinics that provide help to people who have trouble with hoarding as well as providing information about on-line support groups.

- **Address the spiritual component**. How does your faith tradition address deep longings for "enough"? One good book that was recommended to me on this topic lately (albeit around food), was *Made to Crave: Satisfying your Deepest Desire with God, Not Food*. There are many Scriptural passages about depending on God for "enough." Include them in your work with people who struggle with hoarding.

Addressing the deep need to hoard really is a challenging issue, but people can change if they want to. God wants to help. Folks often, however, need the right help.

Health Ministry Advice for Everyone

Loneliness

QUESTION

One of our church members recently confided to me how very lonely she has been since her husband died a few months ago. Are there any health ministry resources or ideas that could be a support to her?

You are right to be concerned. The World Health Organization has identified loneliness as a significant risk factor for illness, particularly among the middle-aged. A recent study of nearly 45,000 people aged 45 and up who had heart disease or a high risk of developing it (published in the Archives of Internal Medicine June 18, 2012), found that those who lived alone were more likely to die from heart attacks, strokes, or other heart-related problems over a four-year period than people living with others. The risk was highest for those aged 45–65, with the risk of early death being increased by 24 percent (versus only 12 percent among those aged 66–80 and no association for those aged 80 or older). Loneliness seems to be very hard on our hearts!

The issue of loneliness is certainly an area that church communities should be able to address. Here are a few ideas for your particular parishioner who is grieving the loss of her spouse.

- **Grief support group.** One important role of a faith community nurse (or a health minister) is acting as a coordinator of support groups. A grief support group is a helpful health promotion activity for a congregation to offer. Contact your local hospital or mental health agencies for the names of counselors or chaplains who might be willing to convene such a group. You might consider partnering with another congregation, too. Or find out if there are already other grief support groups in the area with which folks from your congregation can connect.
- **Bibliotherapy.** Using reading materials is a recognized nursing intervention, and there are a number of good books available on grief to support someone who has lost a loved one. The Rev. Dr. Granger Westberg, the founder of the faith community nursing movement, wrote a seminal book on grief work, called *Good Grief*. Consider forming a book group to discuss this and other helpful books on healing and wholeness.
- **Group service projects.** Is your friend someone who might enjoy working with others on creating a healing garden for the church or the community? Perhaps she is the type who would enjoy participating in a prayer shawl ministry, or a quilter's group.
- **Dinner or lunch group.** Consider asking your friend to participate in a dinner group, This is a great way to get to know other people. Don't try to match her up or have an even number of people. Simply share a meal.
- **Walking program.** Invite your friend to go walking with you. It's hard to be lonely when you are walking with a friend. The data shows that the benefit is two-fold—both social and better health outcomes.
- **Health committee.** Ask your friend if she would be willing to help you by serving with you on a health committee in your church. This would give her the opportunity to minister to others at her own pace, an activity shown to have positive health benefits. This would also get her out and connected with people again.

Don't push, but invite your friend to participate in ways that feel right to her. Don't give up on her, and let her take her time. Your watchful care of her (with notes or calls from time to time) will help her know that she is not alone. Enlist others to help, and soon your friend may be involved again. If not, down the road a bit you may want to help her consider counseling to help her find her social footing again.

Memory Loss Support

QUESTION

We have several parishioners who have developed Alzheimer disease or other forms of dementia. How can we help them and their families?

Few disease processes can be as lonely for a family as watching a spouse or a parent fall into mental decline and fog. There is also growing evidence that a person suffering from dementia has a longer period of awareness, frustration, and distress about the dementia than previously thought, primarily because of problems with speech that mask their true state of cognition.

One relatively new model for providing support for families is called the "Alzheimer Café." Started in the Netherlands in 1997 by Dr. Bére Miesen, this café model offers a monthly themed program for individuals with dementia along with their families and friends. The café offers refreshments, fellowship, networking and high-quality continuing education from health professionals about Alzheimer disease and available community resources. Each Alzheimer Café (AC) meets at a set time, in a set place, with a set format, yet, like a real café, the AC does not require registration and people can come and go as they like.

The Alzheimer Café is a place that can help to reduce the stigma surrounding Alzheimer disease. In the words of Dr. Miesen,

> At the AC dementia is given a status ... Acknowledging (coming out) that "I've got Alzheimer's" or "I've got something to do with dementia" is often the first step on the road to regaining some control, and taking charge of your own life again. By "coming out of the closet" about dementia, you stop yourself from becoming stuck in the role of victim. A good quality Alzheimer Café is a sort of safe haven, guaranteeing the security and assurance needed to enable people with dementia and their families to, as it were, explore the disease and its consequences—both now and in the future, giving them the ability to look their enemy in the eye as quickly as possible. Then they can stop trying to walk away or deny it.

You are right in being watchful and mindful of the potential for elder abuse in your community—is it a global concern. Elder abuse can include physical, emotional, or mental abuse, as well as exploitation, neglect, or abandonment (which may be the case above).

There are 10 such programs across the US at the present time (including a new one at Southminster Presbyterian Church in Beaverton, Oregon, with parish nurse Suzanne VanSlyke), and more than 200 abroad. For more information in English, including a manual on how to set up an AC, visit the website of Alzheimer Café UK.

The Alzheimer's Association is the world's leading partner in providing online and other resources to support people living with Alzheimer disease, along with their families, as well as information for health care professionals and others.

Just one final note: don't underestimate the power of providing respite to family members who are caring for a loved one with dementia. Pick up the phone and check in with them and see how they are doing. Bring them lunch. This is a long journey, and the church can be a critical support along the way.

Elder Abuse

QUESTION

I am worried about one older church member, who lives with her children. She seems to have some strange bruises recently and has been coming to church less often in recent weeks. What can I do?

You are right in being watchful and mindful of the potential for elder abuse in your community—it is a global concern. Elder abuse can include physical, emotional, or mental abuse, as well as exploitation, neglect, or abandonment (which may be the case above).

Elder abuse is a problem that comes with a lot of shame. Who wants to admit that their own children are stealing from them or hurting them in other ways? Who wants to say that their children aren't taking good care of them? Or who wants to admit that they have done things to a parent or another older adult that they never would have dreamed they could be capable of doing?

Not talking about this issue makes the shame feel even greater. Letting people know that this is a concern in communities everywhere—and providing resources to deal with the issue—opens the conversation and encourages people to get the help they need.

According to research at the US Administration on Aging, 1 in 10 seniors may experience abuse, but only 1 in 5 of these situations is reported. In many cases, elders will not be able to speak up for themselves due to a deteriorated physical or mental health condition. In this case, it is the responsibility of extended family and the community (including the medical community and the faith community) to act to protect a senior at risk for, or experiencing, abuse at the hands of another family member, neighbor, or other caregiver.

The National Center on Elder Abuse provides a Help Hotline (a listing for the number is available on their website), a database of state resources for seniors, and information about help for elders and families. If you suspect someone is being abused, call the Help Hotline. Calls to the Help Hotline do not require you to give your name, and you do not need absolute proof to report suspected abuse. (Remember, RNs and other health professionals are mandated reporters, but clergy are not.) If someone is in immediate danger, 911 should be called.

Also, consider inviting a speaker to come to your congregation to make a presentation on this topic. Having someone from the "outside" talk about it raises the visibility, and gives an additional arena for resources to people. A good time might be in preparation for the Annual World Elder Abuse Awareness Day, held each June 15.

To report suspected abuse in a nursing home or long-term care facility, contact your state-specific agency. To find the listing, visit the Long-Term Care Ombudsman website.

Breast Cancer

QUESTION

Someone in my parish was recently diagnosed with breast cancer. How can I support her? Do you have advice on ways the entire congregation might get involved?

There are a number of good ways to support people diagnosed with breast cancer, but not all of them will be helpful for everyone. Some women will want the entire church to support their journey, while others will want only the pastor, parish nurse or a few close friends within the congregation to know. Most women will probably be somewhere in between. This may be even trickier for men who develop breast cancer, which does happen.

Working with a health committee, if your church has one, makes helping a lot easier than letting everything fall to the pastor or to a faith community nurse. One person might coordinate rides for chemotherapy or radiation therapy. Another might coordinate meals to be brought to the person's house on prearranged days. Still another might coordinate a card ministry to send supportive messages along the way.

The faith community or parish nurse, or a trusted and capable friend within the congregation, might (with permission of the patient) accompany the individual to appointments, in order to write down answers to questions and information that the doctor provides so that it can be recalled later. What the doctor says is often forgotten shortly after leaving the office, since so many things are on one's mind. A friendly companion can also make the waiting room time more pleasant and comforting. In addition, the parish nurse or a layperson with medical knowledge can help track down answers to health questions.

Some people will be offended by the pink color used to symbolize breast cancer or the heart pillows, etc. Listen to what they are going through and what they need. Sometimes a support group in the church can be helpful, and other times it is better to find other support groups in the community (hospitals and cancer wellness programs, for example), and to give the person another option. She does not want to be known only as the "breast cancer lady."

Many people living with breast cancer have families at home—spouses, partners, or children—who will be very worried about them, whether or not they are willing to talk about it. Provide an opportunity to care for families, too. Perhaps trusted individuals can offer to provide childcare or pick up a child from school. Grocery shopping, walking the dog—all the normal family activities—are an extra burden at this time and a specific offer of help can really make a difference.

Anyone with breast cancer will want to help others detect it early. Now might be a good time to arrange for a mammography van to come over from your local hospital and offer screenings to the congregation and neighborhood. Often they can be provided free to those without health insurance coverage. And this raises the issue in a non-threatening way for all.

Many people will beat breast cancer. Some will not. Being sensitive in providing support for wherever that person (and her family) is at any given time, will make all the difference in the world.

Grieving Congregations

QUESTION

Grief is a big issue in my church at the moment. Five or six youth in our community have tragically died in the past year and our 53-year-old pastor just unexpectedly died. We invited families who had experienced tragic loss to a special service. What else can we do?

In recent times, when so many have been quickly swept away by tsunamis, floods, and storms, life feels overwhelming. When the unexpected and untimely deaths arrive so close to home, as it has with these devastating losses in your own church and town, people begin to suffer true shock. At this point, it is important to make available all sources of comfort and sustenance, including food and warmth, which you surely already have provided and will continue to provide.

You may want to consider offering healing services on a quarterly, or even monthly basis. Something as simple as a Taizé service can be very comforting, or you may want to offer the option for laying on of hands, blessing, or anointing at services, depending on your denominational traditions and preferences.

Offer times to make the sanctuary available during the daytime and early evening hours for quiet meditation and arrange to have the phone numbers of counselors available. Leave business cards so that people can take them and call at their convenience. Perhaps an elder or deacon could be available for all the times that the church is open, in case someone needs a listening ear.

Depending on how the young people died—suicide or car accidents for instance—you may want to act quickly to provide education to prevent such tragedies in the future, but doing so in a manner that does not further hurt the families who have lost children. For example, in the case of suicide, part of that education must be on ending the stigma around accessing mental health care, and opening up the possibility of talking about mental health issues in the community. Good health information and access to quality health care are key. If you don't have such care available, your church may want to partner with an organization in another town to arrange for a provider to travel to your congregation one evening a week. Talk about whatever has been happening to bring healing and validate the experiences people have been undergoing, as well as to prevent future tragedies.

After-Death Paperwork

QUESTION

Several people in our congregation have died in the past few months. Is there any way we could help their families with the great deal of paperwork that came in the months that followed?

Providing a checklist to families during this time might be of help. Many funeral homes also provide this service. Here are some of the things that people will need to consider (with thanks to the Massachusetts Commission on End of Life Care.) You may want to include these items in your church's newsletter so that people can plan ahead.

- Ask your funeral home to provide at least a dozen copies of the death certificate.
- Notify Social Security that your loved one has died to avoid over-payments. Surviving spouses may be eligible for increased benefits, and minor children may be eligible for benefits as well.
- Contact the employer of your deceased loved one to terminate health insurance coverage for the deceased only, and to ensure that coverage will continue for the rest of the insured.
- Also ask the employer about pension plans, credit unions and union death benefits, if any. Each claim will require a certified copy of the death certificate.
- Contact your life insurance company to file a claim. You will need the policy number and a certified copy of the death certificate to file a claim. Remove the name of the person who died from any policies.
- Return credit cards of the deceased to close those accounts (with a certified copy of the death certificate), or tell the financial institution that you want to remain on the account and keep it open.
- Check with your tax advisor about how to file a tax return for your loved one for the year he or she died.
- Keep monthly bank statements on all individual and joint accounts that show the account balance on the day of your loved one's death. You will need this information for the estate tax return.
- Change any joint bank accounts into your name.
- Change stocks and bonds into your name.
- Assemble all the bills, particularly those that are very important, such as credit cards and mortgages, so that they can be paid on time. Notify each company about the death of your loved one and that your name will be the primary one on the account.
- When you get around to it, notify others such as publications and alumni associations.

Here are the documents you will need to complete these tasks.

- Death certificates (10–20 certified copies)
- Social Security Card
- Marriage Certificate
- Birth Certificate
- Birth Certificate for each child, if applicable
- Insurance policies
- Deeds and titles to property
- Stock certificates and bank books
- Honorable discharge papers for a veteran and/or VA Claim Number (call the Veterans Administration at 800-827-1000 for more information).
- Recent income tax forms and W-2 forms
- Automobile title and registration papers
- Loan and installment payment books and/or contracts

Also, the Church Health Center has a couple of great resources related to end-of-life planning that can help facilitate good discussions around topics similar to this. One is *Taking Care of Business: A Guide for the Discussion of Wills, Healthcare Directives, and Funeral Planning*. The second is a Bible study called, *From Life to Life Eternal: Discussing Death as People of Faith*, which provides biblically based reflections on practical issues such as grief and loss, funeral planning, and legal preparations.

Finally, as you know, grief support groups can be helpful, along with reaching out in love and compassion through cards, calls, and visits in the months that follow to those who have lost loved ones.

Caregiver Support

QUESTION

We have a number of caregivers in our congregation, and our health committee would like to know how to be helpful to them. Can you give us some ideas?

Caregivers in your church are busy, and they are tired, and the statistics above don't even mention the financial stress these family caregivers may live with. You need to provide programs with proven success records that will give them tools to make their busy, stressed lives easier.

One such program is Powerful Tools for Caregivers, an evidence-based program based on the groundwork laid by Dr. Kate Lorig, et al. at Stanford University through their Chronic Disease Self-Management Program. This program focuses on stress management, communications skills, and skills for navigating through difficult decisions. Organizations in more than thirty states now offer this program, and you can see if there is already a program being offered in your area. If not, you might consider becoming a trainer for this program. Grant funding is often available to implement this program, so do inquire of local funders for help.

One great service your congregation could provide to caregivers would be to have a two-hour resource fair with a lunch in between. From 11:00 to noon have someone come in and talk about all the resources available for support and respite to family caregivers of seniors, enjoy a meal at noon, and after lunch have someone talk about the resources available for support and respite to family caregivers of special needs children and younger adults with disabilities. That way everyone could be together for lunch, but no one would need to stay for the whole event.

Good places to look for speakers on the topic of senior caregivers would be:

- Your local Area Agency on Aging. Find a branch in your community through the National Association of Area Agencies on Aging
- Gerontologists and other senior service providers
- Education department of your local hospital
- Social work or psychology department of local university

Good places to look for speakers on the topic of special needs children or disabled younger adults would be:

- Special education department of local school district
- The ARC—National Association for Retarded Citizens
- The National Disability Rights Network
- Education department of your local hospital
- Social work or psychology department of your local university

Pastoral care to caregivers is hugely important, and the entire church can help support a family in a variety of ways:

- Send over frozen meals to be used at the family's convenience, or arrange ahead to deliver a ready-to-serve meal.
- Equip trained congregational members to serve as respite providers to sit with the family member and give the caregiver a break.
- Make short phone calls to bring a word of encouragement. Short visits (please arrange in advance) may also be appreciated.
- Regular notes of support for both family member and caregiver would also be greatly appreciated. You can also stay in touch by e-mail.
- Last, but not least, promise to hold them in prayer.

Notes:

Notes:

Notes:

Notes:

Get Going on the Journey to Wellness
with GET MY PEOPLE GOING!

An expanded and updated version of the popular congregational wellness program developed by the International Parish Nurse Resource Center, with new devotionals by Deborah Patterson, author of *The Essential Parish Nurse*, and additional program materials by the Church Health Center.

Get My People Going! Starter Kit includes:
1 Leader Guide +
10 Participant Guides
$60.00

Regular Price:
Leader Guide: $25.00
Participant Guide: $10.00

Order a starter kit for your congregation today!
www.ChurchHealthCenter.org/Store

Discover how to connect your health and your faith now.

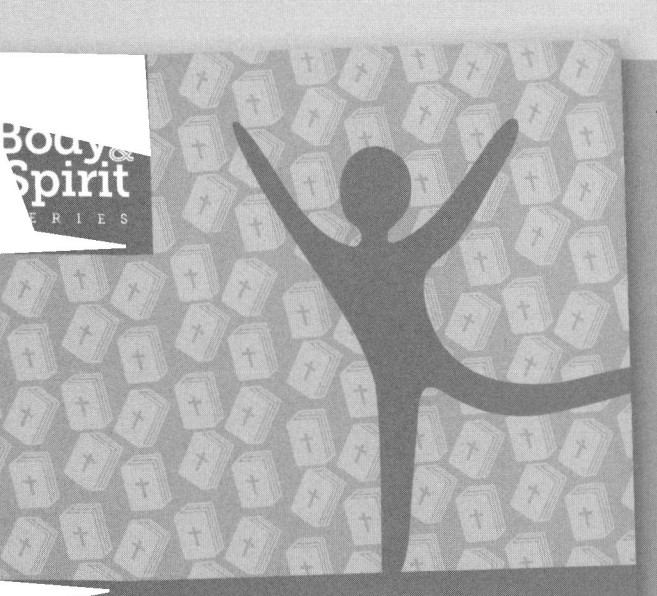

A health class at church? What is that about? It's about engaging with a fundamental dimension of the gospel. Jesus cares about making and keeping people well. Since its early centuries, the church has expressed compassion for the poor through health ministries. More recently, though, we have separated our health and our faith into distinct compartments that rarely intersect.

Jesus said he came so we can have abundant life. In *Body and Spirit: Faith and Health in the Bible*, we explore the gospels to discover the connection between spirituality and wellness. The Bible has a lot to say about this connection.

This is not just a class for health nuts. This is a class for everyone seeking to discover how to connect your health and your faith *now*. Filled with thought-provoking questions, this study will serve as a starting point for conversation about health ministry in your church setting as well as your community.

Body & Spirit:
Faith and Health in the Bible

By Rev. G. Scott Morris, MD
and Susan Martins Miller

www.ChurchHealthCenter.org/Store

"Jill Westberg provides a critically needed step-by-step guide for exploring, designing and implementing health ministries as a team in a congregation, which years of experience have shown to be the most effective and sustainable model for identification and delivery of needed services."
—DEBORAH PATTERSON, author of *Healing Words for Healing People*

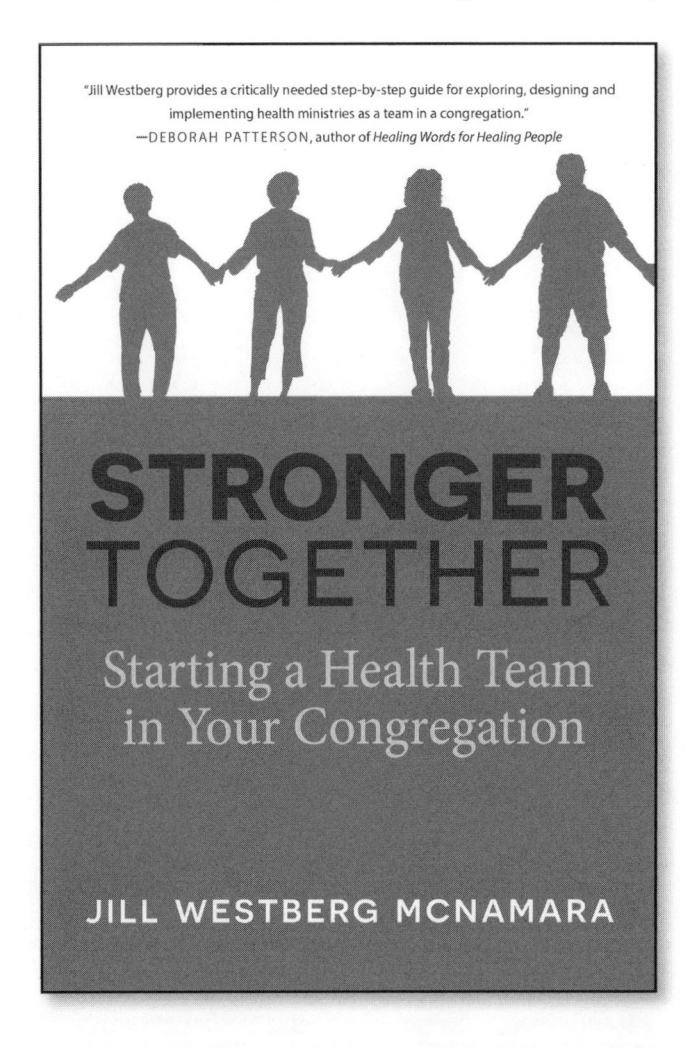

STRONGER TOGETHER
Starting a Health Team in Your Congregation

JILL WESTBERG MCNAMARA

CONGREGATIONS ARE RECLAIMING THEIR ROLE IN HEALTH CARE.
It takes time and determination to develop a health ministry team, but a map through the process can make the route clearer. With a blend of organizational principles, practical tips, inspirational stories, and proven real-life program models in churches, *Stronger Together: Starting a Health Team in Your Congregation* is a valuable guide that your health team—whether just starting out or seeking new energy—will refer to again and again.

www.ChurchHealthCenter.org/Store